Acid Reflux
in Infants and Children

An essential guide for parents, caregivers, and health-care professionals

By

Tracy Davenport, MA and
Mike Davenport, EdD

Acid Reflux in Infants and Children

ISBN: 976-0-9745945-2-1

Produced and distributed by SportWork.
Main Street • P.O. Box 192 • Church Hill, MD • 21623
(410) 556-6030 (phone/fax)
tdavenport@refluxguide.com
www.refluxguide.com

Printed in the United States of America. Cover design by
2econdNature. Editing by Mitchell Editorial Services.

To Brook and Ben

and

to the families who have yet to get help

TABLE OF CONTENTS

PART 3
DISCUSSIONS FROM EXPERTS IN THE FIELD

A PERSONAL NOTE

J ust over a year ago we found ourselves celebrating Christmas and the New Year and giving thanks for the great health care we had finally found for our three-year-old son, Benjamin. Since birth, he has struggled with gastroesophageal reflux and all of the associated repercussions.

The first edition of *Making Life Better for a Baby with Acid Reflux* was published in April of 2004 and has sold around the world to many families experiencing their own struggles with acid reflux. Unfortunately, many of the families who purchased the book wrote to us with horror stories about trying to find adequate health care for their child's condition. So while we were celebrating our own success with building a great health-care team, the struggles of those families were never very far from our hearts and minds.

We had two ideas. Maybe we could help those who, for a myriad of different reasons, did not have access to up-to-date professionals. What if we brought to them the voices of some of those who have helped us? And what if, now that Benjamin is older, we broaden the topic to children instead of just babies?

This book is our response to those two ideas.

Following are three parts that we hope will make an impact. They represent our perspective and the perspective of some of the health-care professionals who are working to make your life better, or your child's life better, or your patient's life better if he or she is a baby or child with acid reflux.

— Tracy and Mike Davenport

CONTRIBUTORS

Susan Bauer, RN, MSN
University of Missouri
Columbia, Missouri

Marcella Bothwell, MD
Assistant Professor
Departments of Otolaryngol-
ogy and Pediatrics
University of Missouri
Columbia, Missouri

Pam Cooper, PhD
Department of Surgery
Applied Research
University of Missouri
Columbia, Missouri

Kim Fincher, DVM
Equine Veterinarian
Chestertown, Maryland

Michele Innes, RD
Alfred I. duPont
Hospital for Children
Wilmington, Delaware

Jeff Phillips, Pharm D
Associate Professor
Department of Surgery
University of Missouri
Columbia, Missouri

Stacy Turpin, MS
Medical Illustrator
Department of Surgery
Applied Research
University of Missouri
Columbia, Missouri

Richard G. Wirtz, PsyD
Chester River Behavioral
Health
Chestertown, Maryland

PART 1

Breaking News Related to Acid Reflux

When we sat down to revise the first edition of *Making Life Better for a Baby with Acid Reflux,* we asked for feedback from some of our contacts. From this feedback, we discovered that we had three main headlines that seem to run throughout the book. We have pulled out all three of them and highlighted them here. You will read more about each of these throughout the book because each of the subjects resurfaces again and again. You will see how important it is to understand these three headlines as you seek treatment for you child with acid reflux.

- ◆ Headline 1: Medicine Today Is Not the Way It Used to Be

- ◆ Headline 2: Reflux Is Frequently Misdiagnosed

- ◆ Headline 3: Medications and New Dosages Are Greatly Impacting Reflux Treatment

Medicine Today Is Not the Way It Used to Be

We live in a rapidly changing world, and the field of medicine is no exception. Not long ago, our parents went to their doctor's office and assumed the physicians knew everything, and that he or she was completely up to date on every illness and treatment. Today, there is such a rapid progression of science and information; no single physician can keep up with all of the advancements. For us, this was headline news. We found a tremendous variability in the knowledge base of physicians when we were seeking treatment for our son with acid reflux and this often translated into how we were treated, and the treatment choices that were offered to our son.

The impact of this medical evolution is so great that we felt this was a critical place to start a book about dealing with an illness such as acid reflux. Following are six areas where medicine has recently changed dramatically.

1. Doctor-Patient Relationship

Medicine is in the new millennium, and with that has come a significant change in the doctor-patient relationship. One place this is most evident is in the decision-making process.

In the past, most health-care decisions were left to the doctors and their staffs and seldom were patients involved in those decisions. Today, many patients expect to be part of their health-care decisions. They want an understanding as to what is happening, and they want involvement in decisions made. As one medical review noted, "Shared decision-making is the rule."[1]

Another place where the doctor-patient relationship has changed is in the expectations of patients. We believe we have higher expectations than our parents had. We also believe that as a society, we are more demanding and outspoken, and we expect things to work right—whether it is the subway, our mp3 player, or our health.

One more place where the doctor-patient relationship is changing is in the requirement of more self-responsibility. With doctors only able to spend 15 minutes at a time with most patients (the average doctor visit ranges from 7–16 minutes[2]) a patient must begin to use more of his or her own knowledge as a guide.

2. Technology Explosion

Computer technology is changing virtually everything, including medicine. In an article in *Wired* magazine, the author noted that, "The coming American health-care system has everything to do with smart cards and dumb terminals, big bandwidth and microprobes, genetic markers and info-markets. And it doesn't look like anything you've read in the paper."[3]

As a result of the recent explosion in technology, there are now many more medical choices, especially in the area of diagnostics and treatment of reflux. For example, our son has had two very different procedures to determine the amount of acid refluxing into his esophagus. Both procedures were pH studies, and both procedures measured the acid in the esophagus, but the similarities stopped there. The important point is not the details of the studies, but to know that there is huge range of diagnostic and treatment choices for acid reflux, and with micro-technology and remote sensing, almost anything is possible.

3. Family Dynamics

The dynamics of the family are also changing the medical community. This becomes clear for so many families living with a baby with reflux. The effect a chronic illness like acid reflux has on a family today may be very different from the effect it might have had in the past. For our parents, taking care of a baby with acid reflux must have been a horrible experience because of limited knowledge of the disease and lack of medications to help. However, back then, there was often a stay-at-home mother or grandmother who could dedicate herself to a baby who was screaming in pain for six months or more.

Now, with the increase in the number of families depending on two incomes and with the pressures that go along with that situation, it is no longer a valid option to placate a parent with an old-fashioned remedy like putting a crying baby on a dryer, or turning on the vacuum cleaner to drown out the noise of a baby in pain. For many families today, there is little nearby familial support, and a greatly reduced cushion in their financial situation. Because of these factors, many parents cannot and will not let a baby suffer. Left untreated, a chronic illness like acid reflux can quickly become a desperate situation.

4. Pharmaceutical Company–Patient Relationship

Revolution in the health-care industry has also been driven by the pharmaceutical companies. Where once the representatives of these companies courted the doctors and their staff, these companies are now speaking directly to the patients through advertisements. You've heard them: "If you suspect acid reflux, talk to your doctor about taking our drug." Or, "Don't forget to ask for the purple pill."

We are inundated with these commercials during breaks in primetime television. These ads often put a lot of pressure on the patients to go to their doctors and demand the medications, and this in turn can put pressure on the doctors to satisfy the patients' requests, whether or not the medicine is the appropriate treatment for the situation.

5. Information Explosion

The Internet has become a powerful and familiar health-care tool. There is now information for consumers/patients on the web about the symptoms and treatment of nearly every type of disease and health condition. Each day, more than 12.5 million health-related computer searches are conducted on the World Wide Web.[4] This means that significant medical information is now available to almost everyone, not just doctors.

Is this a good thing? Tom Ferguson, MD, recently wrote this in an article entitled "The First Generation of E-patients":

> Reports of patients coming to harm as the result of online advice are rare, whereas accounts of those who have obtained better care, averted medical mistakes, or saved their own lives are common. Many e-patients say that the medical information and guidance they can find online is more complete and useful than what they receive from their clinicians.[5]

Another benefit is that e-patients (as patients who are web savvy are often called) can access medical online support groups. These groups have become an important health-care resource, providing emotional support, guidance, health information, and medical referrals for nearly all medical conditions—around the world, 24 hours a day and seven days a week, often free of charge.

6. Alternative Medicine

Medicine is now incorporating what were once scoffed-at options. Alternative types of treatment have recently become more mainstream and respected. Treatments such as chiropractic, acupuncture, and holistic diets are now being looked at as viable methods of care.

So what does this mean for you, a parent of a baby who may have acid reflux? Here are a few thoughts to summarize the significance of this information:

1) All physicians are not created equal when it comes to determining the cause and treatment of your baby's discomfort. You must become a self-directed learner, and find a physician who matches your desired level of involvement in your child's medical care (see Chapter 3).
2) You may be well-served by doing research about your child's illness and possible treatments (see Chapter 2).
3) Part of the discussion of your child's condition should include your family situation (see Chapter 4).
4) Pharmaceutical companies spend billions of dollars a year to try to get you to take their drugs. Up-to-date health-care professionals are your best source of information (see Chapter 13).
5) There is a lot of information out there, often as close as your nearest Internet access (see Chapter 2).
6) Alternative diets and treatments may need to be part of your plan (see Chapters 10 and 11).

1. The Israeli National Institute for Health Policy and Health Services Research. Curriculum for medical schools toward the 21st century, executive summary. The Israeli National Institute for Health Policy and Health Services Research: Jerusalem, Israel. November 18–19, 2002.

2. Creagan, E., and S. Wendel. How Not to Be My Patient: A Physician's Secrets for Staying Healthy and Surviving Any Diagnosis. Deerfield Beach, FL: Health Communications, Inc. 2003.

3. Flower, J. The other revolution in health care. *Wired*. 2.01 (June 1994): 7.

4. Eysenbach, G. The impact of the Internet on cancer outcomes. *CA Cancer J Clin* 53 (2003):356-71.

5. Ferguson, T. The first generation of e-patients. *BMJ* 328 (15 May 2004): 1148-9.

HEADLINE 2

Reflux Is
Frequently Misdiagnosed

One of the heartbreaks associated with reflux is the misdiagnoses many families have to endure before they finally discover that their children suffer from acid reflux. Reflux is a complex disorder and those at the top of the pyramid of understanding know that what was once called "colic" may actually be acid reflux. Those "in the know" also understand reflux symptoms can be much worse at certain times of the day or night, and that reflux can come and go in waves. Health-care providers experienced with reflux also know that parents do not cause their babies to have reflux.

Colic is quickly becoming a fossil term. There are real digestive problems in newborns that until recently were labeled all too quickly as colic. Many providers up to date on the current research now understand that the symptoms of what used to be called colic (pain, long bouts of crying, night awakenings, refusal to eat) can happen for a specific reason, such as acid reflux. Those on the cutting edge are well aware that reflux does not always include projectile vomiting.

Physicians informed about acid reflux in babies and children also know that just like in adults, reflux in babies and children can flare up at the same time of day or night. (Just ask any adult with reflux when the symptoms are the worst. Many will tell you that they feel the worst in the evening, or in the night.) The headliner here is, just because reflux symptoms flare up in the evening, this does NOT make it colic.

Stressed-out mothers and fathers do not cause reflux. However, reflux can certainly stress out mothers and fathers. Taking care of a baby in pain can be extremely distressing. Health-care providers who are well educated about the effort required to care for a baby with reflux will treat you with the utmost respect, and will NEVER blame you for your baby's discomfort.

Does Your Child Have Acid Reflux?
Beyond spitting up, some other symptoms that may be associated with acid reflux are the following:
1) Chronic cough
2) Hoarseness
3) High-pitched sound when breathing
4) Repeated croup
5) Adenoid enlargement
6) Middle ear infections
7) Nose and sinus inflammation
8) Sleep apnea
9) Asthma
10) Sudden Infant Death Syndrome (SIDS)

11)Persistent crying
12)Nighttime awakening
13)Failure to thrive
14)Feeding abnormalities
15)Back arching

The best way to get an accurate diagnosis for acid reflux is with a physician who is familiar with both typical and atypical signs and symptoms of the disease.

Medications and Dosages Are Greatly Impacting Reflux Treatment

M ajor developments in the understanding of acid reflux medications and the dosing requirements of these medications are revolutionizing the management of acid reflux in babies and children. A few specialists in the field are well aware of this knowledge, but many families are not in contact with those individuals.

Of the variety of medications frequently prescribed to treat acid reflux in children some work very well, while there are mixed reviews about others. The breaking news here is that children are not like "little adults" when it comes to many reflux medications. Specifically, it has been found that some children metabolize some medications at a much faster rate than adults, burning through the medication quickly. Dosing requirements to control reflux symptoms in babies and children may require much different dosages than for adults.

Chapter 13, while technical in nature, highlights some of the latest findings about reflux medications.

PART 2

A Parent's Perspective

When a child has acid reflux, an entire family can be affected. Specifically, the effect on the parents can be enormous, from many different angles. With that in mind, the following chapters offer a parent's perspective on what to expect, and actions you may want to consider.

- ◆ Acid Reflux

- ◆ Research for Success

- ◆ Working with the Medical Profession

- ◆ Understand How Hard This Can Be

- ◆ The Baby Isn't Bad: the Pain Is

- ◆ Taking Care of Yourself

- ◆ Money Matters

CHAPTER 1

Acid Reflux

If you are reading this book, something is not right. Something is going on and you need help. Maybe your child is crying for hours, vomiting, or refusing to eat. Or maybe he or she is just plain miserable.

You may know that your child is suffering from reflux as a fact (from a physician) or you may just think or guess he has reflux, and want and need to find answers.

Regardless, acid reflux may be an issue in your life, and we are going to try to help you come to terms with it and get the help you need to improve the quality of your family's life.

At the time we came face-to-face with acid reflux it was just beginning to be truly understood and diagnosed. Gastroesophageal reflux, or GER as it is more officially known, is a normal physiologic process that occurs in healthy infants, children, and adults. Almost all children and adults have a small amount of reflux without being aware of it. When refluxed material rapidly returns to the stomach, it causes no damage to the esophagus. However, in some children, the stomach contents remain in the esophagus and cause damage to the esophagus lining. The stomach contents can also go to the mouth and upper airway and cause a variety of problems.[1]

Signs and symptoms of reflux may include irritability, sudden or constant crying, food refusal, sleeplessness, frequent infections, pneumonia, wheezing, and difficult or painful swallowing, just to name a few.

How Many Suffer?

Each year in the United States, about 8 million babies are born. The estimates of how many babies develop reflux vary, but the high end is approximately 35%. That means as many as 2.8 million babies may show signs and symptoms of acid reflux each year. Of those, about 2%, or 160,000, will develop complications due to the reflux.[2]

Could It Be Colic?

Bluntly, the term *colic* may soon be officially obsolete. Colic has been used to describe pain and discomfort of unknown origin in the abdomen of babies. But now, as the medical profession gets a clearer idea of what is really going on, *colic* may be on its way out and *acid reflux* may well take its place in many cases. We were once told that colic was a five-letter medical term for "we don't really know what is wrong," and from our experiences, we don't doubt it one bit.

What Causes Reflux?

It appears there may be many reasons why stomach contents escape back into the esophagus. It took us about two years to finally learn that the cause of our son's reflux is his allergic reaction to foods that he eats. It seems when Benjamin eats foods outside of his "safe foods," his stomach refluxes. Other children with food allergies may show an allergic reaction by getting hives or asthma, or going into anaphylactic shock. One of Benjamin's reactions is reflux.

Following are some other causes of reflux:

- Immature digestive tract
- Physical defect with LES (lower esophageal sphincter)
- Forces on stomach that cause contents to escape, such as pressure from tight clothes and overeating
- Items that can weaken the LES, such as second-hand smoke or spices
- Disabilities

Treatment

We wish that this section could be a simple paragraph recommending a few steps that would cure your child's reflux. Unfortunately that is not going to happen.

The treatment you find successful for your child may be simple or complex, quick or lengthy. So much of that depends on so many things.

Some common treatments for reflux are the following:

- Time (research suggests most children outgrow reflux by their first birthday)
- Positioning (feeding and sleeping)
- Feeding changes (formula, solids)
- Medication
- Surgery

Reflux is complex and so might be the solution that works for your child. One of the most important steps toward finding a successful treatment may very well be understanding what you are facing. We hope that the next several chapters may provide an insight.

References

1. Bothwell, M.R., D.S. Parsons, A. Talbot, G.J. Barbero, and B. Wilder. Outcome of reflux therapy on pediatric chronic sinusitis. *Otolaryngol Head and Neck Surg* 121 (Sept. 1999): 255-62.

2. Hu, Ze, et al. Mapping of a gene for severe pediatric gastroesophageal reflux to chromosome 13q14. *Journal of the American Medical Association* 284 (July 2000): 325-34.

CHAPTER 2

Research for Success

Simply put, research is the act of seeking truth, information, or knowledge. In the process of trying to get the best treatment for your child with reflux, you are going to have to make a critical decision. You will need to decide how active a researcher you want to be.

At one end of the research continuum is someone like Lance Armstrong, a very active researcher. In a recent article, Armstrong said that education was the key to his survival in his battle with testicular cancer:

> As soon as I saw what I was up against, I began to study the disease and learn everything I could about treatment. I didn't leave it all to my doctors. I became extremely interested—you might even say obsessed—with understanding how the illness affected my body.[1]

At the other end of the continuum is a passive re-searcher who may do nothing more than pick up pam-phlets at the doctor's office.

Reasons to Research

You need to decide where you want to fall in the spec-trum (and where your resources will allow you to go). To help you decide, here are eight possible reasons you may want to research.

Reason #1. GER and GERD are complicated condi-tions. Some medical experts suspect that reflux might actually be several separate diseases. There is a lot of discovery happening about reflux. That means that new information is being published frequently. In the course of your research you might be the one to see something new that sounds very close to your situation and that you may want to discuss with your doctor.

Reason #2. The more you know, the better decisions you can make. Keeping yourself educated on the latest information may make a big difference in your treatment options. For example, even though a doctor that we re-spect very much recommended that we consider major surgery for Ben, our research led us to a very progres-sive group at the University of Missouri that was trying different approaches to the disease. Because of our re-search, we were able to consult with this group as an alternative to surgery.

Reason #3. You can double-check the information that you are receiving from your health-care professionals.

This can be especially helpful when a variety of medications are simultaneously prescribed.

Reason #4. Education can help you speak the same language as your health-care teammates. Understanding the common terminology of GER and GERD can save everyone time.

Reason #5. Research gives you needed confidence in what may be going on. The health-care team we worked with at the University of Missouri recommended that we visit the web site of the pH probe manufacturer. Benjamin was going to have the probe inserted and the Missouri team understood that the more we knew about what they would be doing to Benjamin, the better we would feel about it.

Reason #6. Research might help reduce the emotional edge. A physician only has a limited amount of time to spend with you to explain what may be occurring. By doing your own research you can take as much time as you need to understand what the doctor has told you. In our case this helped reduce our stress.

Reason #7. If you are recommended to a new doctor, research can help you to check the qualifications of the referred physician.

Reason #8. Research can facilitate your understanding of what you will be discussing at your next appointment, and therefore help you to be better prepared to ask specific questions and make better use of the limited time you have with your doctor.

This quote by Beth Anderson, the head of the reflux support group PAGER, might help put the importance of research into perspective for you:

> Unfortunately, changes in the actual treatment of reflux are always a little slower in coming to the public. This is why I always recommend that parents do all they can to educate themselves and keep up with the research that is coming out. Many doctors don't stay current or tend to be wary of the newest treatments but for patients who are not doing well with *older treatments*, it is up to the parents to be constantly on the lookout for promising new ideas.[2]

Cautions

There are also reasons to be cautious if you decide to be an active researcher.

Reason #1. Consider your source. Locating information today is significantly easier than it has ever been, in large part due to the Web. It almost seems as if the information is ready to jump right out at you. You need to take the utmost care when getting any information from the Web, and use only reputable sources. Be mindful that the information is only as reliable as the source.

Reason #2. You can't always generalize. If you are reading studies or reviews of experiments, realize that many findings are not applicable outside of the sample group that was used for the research.

Reason #3. You must use common sense when you get information. We suggest that you use appropriate information you find as material for discussion with your medical team. We strongly, strongly, strongly caution you to not make any changes to your child's treatment or care until you have conferred with your team.

Reason #4. If you are researching, you may be changing your relationship with your physician from the traditional *provider-centered* system to a more *patient-centered* system.

Back in the 1880s physicians did not exist as we know them today. People cared for most of their own health problems, and they had complete access to any and all medical tools and treatments available at that time.[3]

That changed in the 1900s, when a physician-centered health-care system developed. And with that came a dramatic shift with medical tools and treatments becoming the sole property of physicians. This physician-centered ownership kept evolving unhindered until around the late 1960s, when people slowly started to want more control of their health care. This was in part driven by the spirit of those revolutionary years, and also by a crisis in health care due to skyrocketing costs.

This change in ownership was reflected by the seminal book *Our Bodies, Ourselves*, which Dr. Tom Ferguson noted was "the prototype for a new generation of medical guides . . . which would enable them [readers] to play a more responsible role in managing their own health care."

Since then, it seems the change in the doctor-patient relationship has continued to evolve. Ferguson, who is known for his work on the development of online health resources and "e-patients" (http://www.doctom.com), wrote that by the 1990s, "The age of unquestioned 'doctor's orders' has been replaced by an era of 'shared medical decision-making.'"[3]

One of the phenomena we've observed in seeking treatment for our son is that there appears to be a coming collision between a FEW in the medical community who don't seem to understand how readily available medical information is in cyberspace, and those of us who can find just about anything we want on the Web with a wireless connection, a strong cup of java, and about 15 minutes of uninterrupted time. Mix that research capability together with a little old-fashioned thinking about a woman's place in this world, and you can be in big trouble if you aren't aware of the potential for conflict. Just a word to the wise…

And finally, keep this one thought in mind:

If something sounds too good to be true, it probably is.

So often, people buy things or try things because they believe that there is a miracle cure handy. Seldom does that ever work out well.

TOOL #1: Doing Research

Knowledge is power. The following steps can help you gain valuable information about your situation.

Needed: Telephone, access to the Web, note-taking material, library access.

There once was a fisherman who made his living by going out each morning, casting his net into the ocean, and bringing his catch back to sell at the dock. He made a good living because he knew four things. First, he knew *why* he was fishing. Second, he knew *what* type of fish people were going to buy each day. Third, he knew *where* he could find those fish on a specific day. And fourth, he knew *how* to fish.

Before you begin any quest for information, think of yourself as that fisherman. Your quest will be much more productive if you know: (1) why you are looking for information, (2) what knowledge you are looking for, (3) where the best place is to find the information, and (4) how to find it.

Let's take a closer look at the why, what, where, and how of researching reflux and GERD.

Step 1: Why and what? The *why* is fairly simple: you are trying to improve the quality of life for you, your child, and your entire family. Exactly *what* information you are looking for is going to be a little bit harder to determine because that may change on a day-to-day basis, not unlike what fish people are buying. For instance, one day you may want to know something like, "What exactly is a Tucker Sling?" and the next day you might want to know "When will this all get better?" Pin down your *what* before you begin researching. It will keep you from getting overwhelmed and sidetracked.

Step 2: Where to look. Now we're getting to the tricky part. Where do you turn for answers to your *what*? We have identified seven sources of information that we use. Here they are in alphabetical order:

- ◆ Articles
- ◆ Friends in the medical community
- ◆ Friends/family with reflux
- ◆ Parents of other children with reflux
- ◆ Studies
- ◆ Support groups
- ◆ Websites

Each one of those areas has given us a wealth of information that has helped us improve the quality of Ben's and our lives. Table 2-1 lists some examples of this information.

Table 2-1. Examples of Available Information

From this source:	We learned such things as:
Articles	The lay person's view of GERD and reflux.
Friends in the medical community	To push hard to find solutions.
Friends/family with reflux	That the pain can be horrific, that reflux keeps many people awake much of the night, that a drink of water can help immensely during an episode.
Parents of children with reflux	That certain foods may make reflux worse, that reflux can cause many other problems (e.g., asthma).
Academic studies	The medical and experts' view of GER and GERD.
Support groups	So many other parents were sharing our experiences.
Web sites	Potential reaction to some medications, research that our medical team was involved in.

Step 3: Now for the *how*. We tend to be very simplistic in our research, in that we basically have broken the *how* down into two methods: We ask questions and we read a lot.

Ask questions. A very important part of research that many folks overlook is that of asking questions. We have asked, and probably will continue to ask until Benjamin is cured, an enormous number of questions. And interestingly enough, the answers to those questions often lead to other questions whose answers can be critical.

For instance, we were discussing Ben's condition with a friend who happened to be a pathologist. Her child had reflux. Very early into Benjamin's illness we told her that he had been diagnosed with *colic*, and asked her what would she do, if this was her child. Her words still ring in our ears today. She said, "Well, I wouldn't stop there!" That advice prompted us to find out more, and we found out that Benjamin had *GERD*, which we had never heard of before. And that advice stayed with us through the entire process. One simple question delivered an answer that had a major impact.

Read. A few years back we were browsing through a used book store. We came upon a book entitled *How to Read a Book*. After initially scoffing at the title, we opened it up, and we've got to say, it's a good book—really good—and they have sold a multitude of copies of it since its original printing in 1940.

So what does that have to do with reflux research? Well the authors, Adler and Van Doren, identified three types of reading: reading for entertainment, reading for information, and reading for understanding. The authors noted that doing research using the last two types of reading is the most effective.

Reading for information and/or understanding is an active process. Reading for entertainment is passive, and many folks get into difficulty when researching when they try to research like they read for entertainment. Basically, how you skim the *TV Guide* doesn't work well for reading scientific articles.

Look at it this way, when you are researching, you are trying to gain information from people who know more than you. If you asked a person a question, he or she would usually give you an answer—pretty easy. However, when you read with a question in mind you must answer it yourself, and that takes work. Today, most scientific writings are written for experts by experts. That means you really have two choices when researching.

The first choice is *scientific popularizations*, such as magazine and newspaper articles. The information in them is usually presented in an easy-to-read manner, which might make digesting the material easier. While these are great beginner researching resources, you will be at the mercy of reporters who filter the information for you.

The second choice is *scientific articles*. These are often dry and lengthy. However, reviewing the articles and focusing on the abstract and discussion sections may offer you some valuable insight. Also, a review of the reference section might be enlightening.

One very important part of reading for research is note-taking. We're not going to get into that here, but let us say that if you read something applicable or of interest then you should write it down because it can easily disappear. Another important part is to achieve an understanding of what you are reading before you begin to criticize or assess significance.

Finding items to read shouldn't be difficult—the nearest source of medical literature is really no farther away than a computer with an Internet connection. Here is an example of how to do it:

1) Find a computer with Internet access and go to http://www.google.com.
2) In the "search" box, type in the signs that you are observing in your child. For example, you might put in "crying," "choking," and "spitting up."
3) Hit return. You will probably see pages and pages of information. Just scan this information, knowing that as you gain more information about your child's condition, some of these articles may become more meaningful.
4) Read away. But remember, be cautious of the source you are using.
5) To further fine-tune your research, click on the "Advance Search" button, and follow the guidelines. Try a variety of key words such as "acid reflux," "colic," "vomiting," and "gagging," and see what you get.

6) Be aware that rarely will you find the full text of a medical article on-line; instead, comprehensive summaries are often offered. If you find a "must-have" article, then take the specific reference information to your nearest library and request a copy of the article.

7) See the end of the book for a more specific list of resources.

References

1. Armstrong, L. Winning the race against testicular cancer. *Vitality* 2 (2005): 12-13.

2. Anderson, B., and L. Anderson. Practical hints on caring for babies with reflux. (Unpublished manuscript, 1992).

3. Ferguson, T. What e-patients can teach us about health care reform. *E-Patients, Online Health, and the Search for Sustainable Healthcare.* (White paper funded by the Robert Wood Johnson.) Forthcoming.

CHAPTER 3

Working with the Medical Profession

H ere we are three years after Ben was diagnosed with reflux and it is time for us to have a real heart-to-heart conversation with you. Before we begin, though, we want you to know that this chapter was a terrific challenge for us to write because we were really conflicted—almost like we were wearing two hats.

The first hat sits on a set of parents who are cool, calm, and collected, writing on a computer while our two children play nicely in the next room thanks to an incredible medical team. Gratefully, this team has gotten our youngest to a point of stable health.

The other hat sits on a set of parents who are incredibly upset and frustrated at how difficult it was to get to this point—the point of having a medical team who really understands the complexity of acid reflux. And our frustration goes beyond our own family. We are also angry about the stories we have heard since our first book, about the difficulties others have had in their search for a good medical team.

Just as an example, one parent in Michigan wrote,

> My first child was very fussy, but my second is different. My pediatrician has been completely unhelpful and condescending, and I can't get in to the pediatric gastroenterologist's office for months.

Another caregiver from New Jersey sent this message:

> I am so sad and feeling pretty unsupported by those who are supposed to have my son's best interest at heart. I have some doctors' names who are supposed to be good, but let's face it—all I really want is someone who will LISTEN to us!

When we hear stories like this we realize that no one is benefiting from these situations, especially the patients. In Chapter 8, Dr. Fincher reminds us that the practitioners often have only a short and swift acquaintance with the patient, and suggests that in most cases the families being cared for are the authorities of their own health care. But when you find a doctor who will listen (Figure 3-1), stick with her.

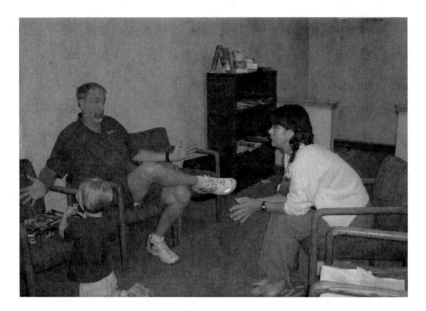

Figure 3-1. Dr. Marcy Bothwell of the University of Missouri
listening.

And this is the nature of our heart-to-heart with you. The
bottom line is this: the medical community works for you
and your family. Seriously, the medical community works
for YOU! And they need to listen to you.

It absolutely amazes us how this very simple concept
has become so convoluted. Some patients are under the
impression that they should blindly go along, unquestion-
ingly, with a doctor's orders, for no other reason than
because, well, because they are ordered by a doctor.
We are here to tell you: not quite, especially for families
of infants and children who suffer from acid reflux.

Acid Reflux in Infants and Children

When you hire health-care professionals, you are selecting a medical team to help you get your child better. To use a sports analogy, you are the owner of a sports team, and your primary doctor is the coach. He or she will call the plays; yet in the end, you will have the final say.

Here is one situation we experienced in which the doctor forgot who was the client (who was working for whom). We had just taken Benjamin to the hospital for an evaluation, and in preparing for the visit we read as much as we could find on reflux and the medications Benjamin was taking. During the visit, the physician at the hospital came in to look at Benjamin and we began to ask him questions. You could tell he was put off by our questions, which were simple and politely put. Finally, in frustration he looked at us and told us, "Stop reading so much. Leave it to us!"

In essence he told us to shut up and do as we are told. What would you do if you took your car to a mechanic, and he came back and told you that you had this major problem? You then begin to ask him a few questions and he tells you to "just do as I say and stop asking questions!"

New mechanic? You betcha.

Our point is that we believe that the patients have the right to define their own reality, and their voices should be heard in their accounting of their own situation, especially relative to taking care of a baby with reflux.

You see, caring for a baby who has acid reflux is different—so very different—from caring for a healthy child for two very significant reasons.

First, reflux is a complex illness, just now beginning to be somewhat understood, involving patients who in many cases cannot be helpful in treatment because they cannot yet talk, and the emotion can be so high and the discomfort so intense.

Second, caring for a child with a chronic illness is often like being submerged into a strange new world of doctors and hospitals. For example, imagine that you've just been hired for a new job. You like it and it is fun and hard work at the same time, and you're doing well. Then one day the boss walks in and says, "Listen, we're going to make a change here with your job description. First off, I want you to work with the group on the 17th floor. Now I know that they speak a different language, but you can learn it. And I know that they are only around every so often and they are incredibly busy, so you'll need to make appointments days if not weeks in advance to see them. And don't be surprised if you have to wait a long time in their waiting room before your appointment. And when they do see you they very well may give you conflicting information, based on their training and experience.

"Also in this new job you may need to travel and stay in strange places, maybe for days at a time, and you might end up sleeping in a chair or on a window sill in a hospital room. And at the same time you are trying to figure this all out, you will have to comfort your baby who is most likely having a horrible time—trouble eating, or sleeping, or both. Oh, yeah, and all of this happens immediately. Right now."

That in essence is what happens when your child has reflux. Life is moving along nicely, then suddenly you find yourself immersed in a strange new world, an unusual place where the language, rules, and expectations are so different.

That is exactly what happened to us. Before we knew it, terms such as *esosphogitis*, *pH levels*, and *proton pump inhibitors* became part of our dinner conversations. We were spending hours in doctors' offices where rules really are different than in the outside world. For example, we encountered one doctor who complained that we called too frequently when we observed our son having episodes of apnea—during which he would stop breathing. Needless to say, we couldn't find the manual anywhere that described how often you *should* call the doctor when your child stops breathing.

What To Do?

So what should you do? What is the best way for you to work with the medical profession?

Our hope is that the following points will help you find the best medical team possible and become an effective advocate for your child. While each of the points could be a chapter in itself, we are counting on the fact that if you have the resources to be reading this book, then a word to the wise will be sufficient.

Take charge. If your child has reflux, your child is ill. Every time he screams, he is saying, "HELP ME!" He needs an advocate, someone to campaign for him, to find out what is wrong. In the beginning of the process, this person is you.

Here is what we mean by taking charge. There is information that will be needed—*you* will have to get that. There will be appointments that will have to be juggled— that's *your* responsibility. You might have to, want to, or need to travel to get the best care—that's on *your* shoulders. And all the while you will need to keep your life in balance.

Hire the best. The best people will do the best work, so why not have the best on your team? It seems to us that often patients aren't overly selective about their health-care providers.

Time and time again during our research we found testimony from parents of infants and children with reflux who were having a difficult (or impossible) time with their doctors. Now, we know that there are many, many good doctors out there, working long and hard to help, like in this example:

> From the moment I entered the specialist's room on that day, this story took a significant turn from [my other child]. Not only was I believed, but I was asked my opinion, and we discussed the possible causes, treatments, and options open to me, and

> then he simply asked what I wanted him to do and we discussed it. At all times, I was the one that was given the choice of what was to be done and the direction in which we should head. I came out of that room feeling informed, in charge of the situation, and thus empowered to handle it.[1]

However, there are also some doctors working in the field, who, like the following example, can make things so much more difficult than they need to be:

> On the fourth day, my Maternal and Child Health Nurse visited. "You need to relax." Lucas (the baby) continued to scream. On the fifth day, the visiting nurse told me that all babies cried! "But he is screaming," I protested. "There's something wrong." "You're doing fine," she said. On the sixth day, I went to my doctor. "All babies cry," he said. "Try to get some sleep." When I protested that Lucas only slept in 30-minute cycles and only 7 of them in 24 hours, he said, "That is normal, it will get better." It didn't![2]

To insure that you're hiring the best, check the credentials of the doctor(s) that you are going to work with. It is not so important that you ask where they went to medical school, or where they did their residency, but it is really important that you find out about their experience with reflux in infants and children. Find out if there are any current patients you could talk to for a reference (this may be difficult due to patient confidentiality issues, but a reflux support group might be able to help). Ask people whose opinion you hold in high regard whom they might recommend. Do some homework, and then hire the best you can.

Blend information. Sometimes you will know things the experts don't. With Benjamin, since we were with him all the time, we knew his sleeping and eating patterns, we knew what his different cries meant, and we got to the point where we could almost predict when he would re-flux. Compare this to what a physician observes seeing him for a brief time, maybe 15 to 30 minutes a visit. There was obviously some information we knew that the rest of the team didn't.

On the other hand, there was a lot that the medical team knew that we didn't. With that in mind, what we would do was blend and share the information to try to get the most complete picture of Benjamin's health that we could.

Look for ideas in unusual places. The solutions for reflux are not necessarily simple. Between what you know about your baby and what your medical team knows about GER and GERD, a solution may be at hand . . . maybe. Often solutions, especially concerning some of the finer points of GERD, may not be found on a short and simple path. For instance, we received some excel-lent advice from our lawyer and his wife who had an in-fant with reflux. Our chiropractor and pharmacist also had wonderful insights, along with our dentist. They helped us see patterns and ask questions that helped us clarify our thoughts. Even our veterinarian was helpful. He reminded us of the importance of the voice of the caregiver who is caring for those who cannot speak.

Just be careful about the information you receive since sometimes it might not be appropriate or even healthy. So be prudent, and check any ideas with your medical team, and be extremely cautious about questionable sources of information on the Internet.

Communicate clearly. This is absolutely critical when working with the medical profession, yet few folks communicate well—especially when they are sleep deprived and are reacting to their baby's suffering. In a doctor's office, where time is very limited, and conversations are often brief, each word counts. If you find that your current level of frustration and exhaustion (or any other factor) will prevent you from communicating clearly, try something simple like having a friend make notes of his observations of what is going on and present them to the physician, or bring the friend with you to the appointment. This bit of objectivity might help clarify to the physician what is happening.

Remember that communication is a two-way interaction. Be sure to listen carefully and be very detail oriented. Take notes at each of your appointments since a great amount of information is often covered in a short amount of time, while you are trying to hold an impatient patient! *Set realistic expectations.* One of the early expectations we had was that Benjamin would get healthy quickly. That turned out to be overly optimistic. Even as

Ben celebrated his first birthday, reflux was a very big part of his and our lives.

Another expectation we had was that we would be able to get the answers to our questions quickly. However, that did not happen because the doctors were often under pressure with regard to their time, and the answers were not always obvious.

We quickly learned a good approach was to tell the doctors that we had questions regarding our child's diagnosis and treatment, and asked them how and when they would prefer that we ask those questions. We followed up that question with one asking what would be a realistic time frame to expect our answers.

Improve yourself. Most people work daily to improve themselves. They do homework, read, solve problems, and do other assorted things to get smarter. Why is it then when faced with a situation like a medical problem, many parents fold up? Why do they forget all of their educational training? It is important that you educate yourself daily about your baby's health.

Know yourself and your medical team. Be true to yourself and be who you are. For example, if you are an assertive person, and that puts your medical team on edge, or the team doesn't respond well to you, then you need to change your medical team. Or if you are a mild-mannered person, and you feel that you are being uncomfortably pushed, then make a change. Be aware of what is going on and be true to yourself.

Advocate for your people. Dr. Fincher has made her living advocating for beings who can't speak, who can't use words to express their pain, their discomfort, their problems.

Your job is no different than hers when you are the parent of an infant with reflux. Babies can't use words to communicate, so they cry. (Our three-year-old is just now able to tell us he has "icky stuff" in his throat.) You need to take your child's communication and turn it into words that others can understand so you can be an advocate for your child.

Be adaptable. Part of being a parent is being adaptable. You invited a new person into your life. That means extra jobs to do and a lot more work. Magnify that five- or ten-fold when you have an infant with reflux.

We've found over the last few years that our life is one of continually being flexible. At a moment's notice our plans may change, because Ben gets sick or we need to do things to keep him healthy.

Letting go. There will probably come a point in your search for the best health care for your baby that you'll need to let go. You will have to trust your medical team or other advisors. If you've done all your homework this will hopefully feel right.

One of the times that really hit us was when a doctor heard something in Benjamin's lungs and he wanted to check for aspirations, to rule out pneumonia. So they said they wanted to take a chest x-ray. This is the first time we had ever been through that process and we said, "Sure, no problem." We both had had x-rays before, and compared to some of Ben's other testing, we thought the x-ray would be simple. Not quite.

With an infant, a chest x-ray is dramatically different. They don't just lie on a table. They are put on a seat in a bike-like contraption, and the poor child, with arms above head, is squeezed between two pieces of round plastic, unable to move. It looks like the worst carnival ride that you can imagine and seeing our screaming infant in there stopped our hearts (Figure 3-2).

So here is Ben screaming as loud as he could, frightened to death, and we had to trust. We had to let go. And so we did, and luckily the test showed no pneumonia.

Take care of the details. Appointments, payments, and paperwork: three critical details. Oftentimes as a caregiver you are asking a group of professionals to go beyond their usual call of duty. Be fair with them. Make sure that you are keeping up with your payments and any other behind-the-scenes tasks.

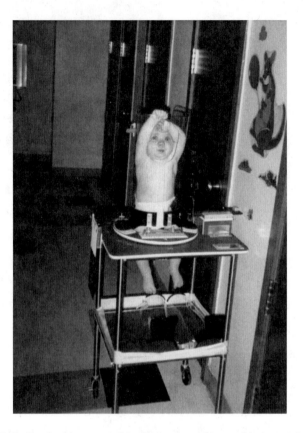

Figure 3-2. Benjamin preparing for a chest X-ray. He is enclosed in a plastic tube that forces his arms above his head.

Respect. There needs to be mutual respect between you and the medical team. You have to respect the doctor. He or she must be able to intervene if things are not going well, and that is truly what is meant by being "under a doctor's care."

There may be a time when your doctor recommends something that you are not comfortable with at first. At that point it will come down to trust and respect (and what the latest research says) as to whether or not you take his or her advice.

After many months of inadequate medical care, our *new* pediatric gastroenterologist, at Georgetown University, wanted to admit Ben to the hospital for further testing. While we were terrified of further heartache, from all accounts this doctor was wonderful, and we needed to trust him. As it turned out, with his help, he was able to pinpoint the severity of Ben's reflux and to refer us for further consults.

This respect is a two-way process. Most worthy doctors will realize that for you to have made it this far with this situation, you must be an exceptional parent. That doctor will also know that because you are with that child more than anyone else, you have information that the other team members don't have. They need to respect you and not be threatened by an inquisitive parent who is working hard to help his or her child.

Just keep in mind that respect should not be confused with abdication. Respect means that you listen and regard someone as a professional. Respect does not mean that you blindly go along, fearful of questions, afraid to voice your opinion, unwilling to get the answers you need.

Have a good sense of humor. More than likely you'll have some dark nights and days ahead of you. As a parent, finding humor when and where you can might make things a little better.

Evaluate. Evaluating how things are progressing with your baby's treatment is a simple step that quite often is not done, yet it is critical in terms of seeing if your medical team is on track and your baby is getting better.

Here is what we did whenever we began a new course of treatment for Ben. We would do an assessment before the treatment and then again after the treatment (or after a period of time). We evaluated if things had improved.

For example, one benchmark we would use is how Ben slept at night. There was a period of time when Benjamin would wake up every 20 minutes, and was only sleeping about 5 to 6 hours per day—total. So when we began a new treatment we made sure that we had solid records of his pre-treatment sleep. And then we tracked again after two weeks or so. In this case, by a change of medications, we saw a great improvement in his sleep. So our evaluation showed that we were on the right track.

When you evaluate, use objective criteria (facts) like how many times the baby vomits per day, how many ounces he eats, or how many times he wakes up during his sleep—objective criteria that can help you evaluate. For example "woke seven times" is more factual than "slept poorly," and "cried one hour" is more specific than "was miserable." Tool #2, at the end of this chapter, may be helpful.

Make more than one appointment. Appointments, appointments, appointments: odds are good that there are going to be a heck of a lot of doctors' appointments popping up on your calendar. That means someone needs to be responsible for organizing them, and don't underestimate how critical this job will be. In one ten-day period we had ten doctors' appointments. That took an enormous amount of juggling between our work schedules, our other son's schedule, and life as a whole to make it work.

Speaking of appointments, we need to make this specific recommendation:

> *MAKE AN APPOINTMENT FOR TWO*
> *DIFFERENT DOCTORS IN TWO*
> *DIFFERENT PLACES IF YOU ARE*
> *REFERRED TO A SPECIALIST!*

(If you think that when you see something written in all capital letters that person is yelling, well . . . you're correct in this instance. We are yelling this recommendation, as loud as the print on this page will let us.)

Here is why you should make two appointments. Getting in to see these professionals can take months and months. Believe us, we know that getting in to see any specialist will seem like a relief to you and your family. However, you want to protect yourself in case a referral doesn't work out.

Unfortunately, there are some medical professionals who not only don't know about reflux and GERD, some of them will even "fake it" and dispense bad information and maybe even bad medications or a bad diagnosis. You don't want to have the misfortune of waiting a very long time to get in to see someone like this.

For instance, we were working with a GI nurse at a teaching hospital and were describing to her the terrible sleeping problems that Benjamin was having. Her response was, "I've never heard of reflux keeping anyone awake before." (When we finally did get good help and related that story to another GI nurse at another teaching hospital, her reply was, "What planet was she from?")

Yet another reason to make more than one appointment is that it happens occasionally that, when a child isn't thriving and the doctors don't have a firm answer, they start blaming the mother or the father. If you have any inkling that this might be happening to you, grab your diaper bag and run for the door as quickly as you can. By having two appointments you won't have to wait another three months to see someone else.

With two appointments, you can always cancel the second appointment if you sense that the first doctor is right on track with helping your child.

Get and give information. A common scenario is that when your child begins to first show signs of reflux you go to your family doctor. If your family doctor needs more information on diagnosing and treating he may send you to a pediatrician. If the pediatrician needs more information, she may send you to a specialist such as a gastroenterologist. If the gastroenterologist needs more information he might send you to an allergist; a respiratory specialist; or an ear, nose, and throat specialist for tests.

The above illustration is one way in which a physician might get more information about a patient's illness. However, it is not nearly as clear-cut for parents of these special babies how they get information. But there are several things that you can do.

Hit the road. You may have to travel to get the best care for your child, but it may be well worth it. In the course of Ben's care it was necessary for us to go to five different hospitals in four different states. Too much time with a misdiagnosis just adds to heartache and unnecessary fatigue. Find where the best doctors are and go there. Don't settle for second best just because it is closer to home. We did one time and it almost destroyed our family.

Another reason to travel is that different places may use different technology in diagnosis and treatment of reflux. Figures 3-3 and 3-4 show two different types of pH probes that were used on Benjamin to diagnose the severity of his reflux. In one test we had to stay in a hospital setting while the test was conducted. The other photo shows a remote sensing pH probe that allowed us to leave the hospital during the test. As you can see, there is a happy boy in only one picture.

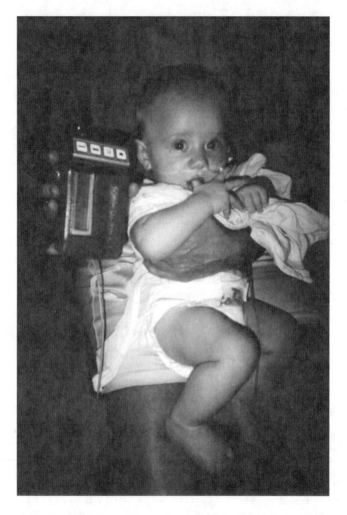

Figure 3-3. A conventional two-channel pH probe requiring a hospital stay.

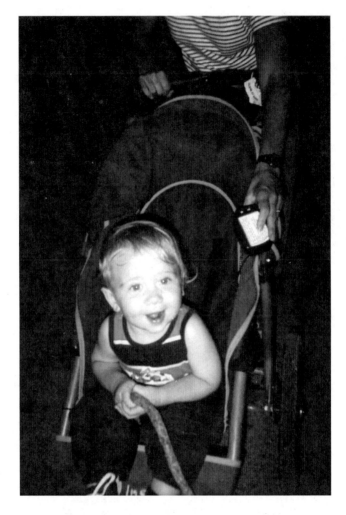

Figure 3-4. A remote sensing pH probe at
University of Missouri--Columbia, done as out-patient, allowed us to
leave the hospital.

TOOL #2: Are You And Your Medical Team Working Well Together?

The following should help you assess whether you and your medical team are working well together.

Determining how well things are going with your medical professionals can be problematic for several reasons. First, if you have an ill child, this is probably a fairly emotional time for you—and that can cloud judgment and make communication difficult. Second, some medical professionals have a tough time relating to parents (especially upset parents) about what may seem like simple issues such as sleeping and eating. Third, some medical professionals are biased by their own research—causing them to make biased judgments. For instance, if a physician is researching behavioral issues, then that doctor will probably be more prone to suspect behavioral causes over mechanical causes.

In a recent issue of the PAGER newsletter, Dr. Sears, a noted pediatrician, wrote about this specific topic:

> I would see babies six and nine months old who had been to four or five different physicians. "Colic," "Worried Mother," "overreactive," all kinds of misdiagnoses. The worst I heard was letting the baby cry it out. I had mothers come in and we would do an esophagoscopy and find ulcers practically burned through the baby's esophagus wall. The poor moms had been told to let the

baby cry it out because they were "spoiling" the baby.[3]

You don't want that to be you, so how do you find out if things are going favorably with your medical team, since that actually is not the type of question that you ask someone point-blank?

Here are a few suggestions to help you tease out the answer.

Suggestion 1: Research. There are three important parts here. First, is your health-care team up on the current research? Do they know about current trends, studies, and types of treatments? How can you find out if they are? Well, you can ask them. That's one way. Another is to compare their recommendations, treatments, and prescriptions to those from other doctors (support groups can help with this).

Second, do they support you as a member of the team? As we note in the previous chapter "Research for Success," many patients or parents are doing a significant amount of their own research about their child's illnesses. To them this is an important part of their healing process. Other patients don't care to do their own research, which is a personal choice. So, does your health-care team support the role that you need to play in getting your child better?

Third, is your health-care team doing its own research that might be a conflict of interest? For instance, a physician who is treating a child with a complicated illness, and who may also be receiving grant money to investigate a type of child abuse such as Munchausen Syndrome by Proxy (MSBP), may not have your best interest at heart. In other words, if they are researchers, make sure their area of research is focused on healing the child, not blaming the caregiver.

Suggestion 2: Are you better off? There is one telltale item that can really give you an insight how things are going. Answer this question, and you'll have your insight:

> Is the quality of my life, and my child's life, better <u>now</u> than it was <u>before</u> we began working with our current health-care team?

When Benjamin turned seven months old we asked that exact same question. The answer came from both of us at exactly the same time . . . a no-hesitation no-doubt-about-it "NO!" Benjamin's quality of life was much worse and so was ours, and it seemed to be getting worse almost weekly. It was at that point that we made a health-care team change. Now we ask that question almost weekly, and we are blessed because so far the answer has been a rousing "YES!"

Suggestion 3: Gut check. If neither of the previous suggestions offers any insight, try this: do a *gut check*. In sports we use that term to signify when an athlete has reached a point in training or competition when he or she must assess if things are right on track. Well, you do the same, and listen to the answer.

So ask yourself, "Are things on track? Do I feel that my health-care team is working favorably for me and my family?" And as we said, listen to the answers.

TOOL #3: Gathering Data about Your Child's Reflux

The following steps, along with Form 3-1 should help you track important information about your child's illness.

Knowledge is power, and that saying is so truthful when it comes to the signs of your child's reflux. (A *sign* is an observed indication of an illness, as compared to a *symptom*, which is an indication felt by the patient.) The more you know about the signs, the better care you can give to your child and get for your child. This task is designed to help you gather some objective knowledge in what is probably a very emotional and difficult time. The steps are simple, but don't underestimate how powerful this information can be.

For us, knowing the signs made a critical difference in Benjamin's care. He was exhibiting many of the classic signs of reflux (arching, screaming, food refusal, multiple awakenings, vomiting). Once we started tracing those signs, patterns became apparent. From that information we learned that certain foods seemed to increase the signs. We also noticed that different positions, such as holding or sleeping (Figure 3-5) made a difference in the number and severity of signs. And we began to see that some of the medications prescribed for Benjamin actually were making him sicker.

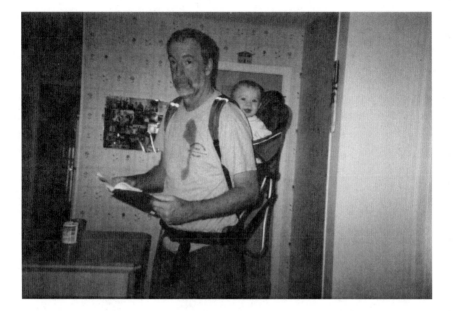

Figure 3-5. Benjamin seemed to do best in an upright position. However, before we could get him in the backpack he refluxed on his dad.

You are the ones who are observing your child day and night. In most cases the doctors will only see your child for a small window of time, and doctors have running through their head massive amounts of published bio-logical and medical literature, and are usually extremely busy.

Step 1: Prepare to track. You need to track your child's signs, so get ready. You'll need a tracking sheet, writing utensil, and a plan for tracking.

Step 2: Get a form. We've included on the next page a sample form we made to track Benjamin's signs. If you want to copy it directly from this book, you can; you just might need to set the copier to an enlarged size to make the copy more user friendly. We use (we often still track) one form per day. If you want to make your own form, try this . . .

Step 3: Do it yourself. If you are computer literate, and you have Excel or any other spreadsheet program, it should take you about 10 minutes to make a tracking-form template. The most difficult part for us was to figure out exactly what items we wanted to track. This took about two weeks of trial and error, and as you can see on our form, we really got down to the basics.

We suggest that you include a 24-hour axis, so that you can note when the signs occurred. Additionally, we recommend that you note the exact time when you give medications. This step is important for two reasons. First, you might see patterns emerge related to the medications and the signs. Second, you really need to know when you give medications.

This can be critical because some medications need to be given at a specific amount of time before meals and some at a specific amount of time after meals. But that really is secondary to the fact that if your child is ill

Form 3-1. Tracking chart

TIME →	3 A	4 A	5 A	6 A	7 A	8 A	9 A	10 A	11 A	12 P	1 P	2 P	3 P	4 P	5 P	6 P	7 P	8 P	9 P	10 P	11 P	12 A	1 A	2 A
SLEEP																								
VOMITING																								
MEDS #1																								
ARCHING																								
MEDS #2																								
PAIN EPISODE																								
CHOKING																								
SNEEZING																								
FOOD																								

enough to be on medication you are probably sleep deprived or at least just distracted. If you are, you need to take steps to ensure you are giving the proper dosage. This is really important when more than one person might be giving the medications.

Step 4: Collect and copy. When you start accumulating forms, make a copy of them for your own records, and store them away in a safe place. Then, at your next doctor's appointment, take the originals in and discuss them with your health-care team. Especially note to them any trends you've noticed.

To assist you in taking charge, the previous form will give you a format to record information and observations to present to your health-care provider in an objective manner.

References

  1. Rebecca's story. *Reflux Digest* 6:1 (summer 2002): 7.

  2. Lucas's story. *Reflux Digest* 5 (spring/summer 2001).

  3. Staff writer. Interview with Bill Sears, M.D. *Reflux Digest* 6:1 (Summer 2002): 4.

CHAPTER 4

Understand How Hard This Might Be

I f you have a baby with acid reflux you are about to embark on a journey that could be more intense than anything you have ever undertaken. We are going to offer you a parent's perspective in this chapter. Dr. Wirtz, an expert on working with families with chronically ill family members, will offer a psychologist's perspective later in the book.

This part comes from us, parents who have been in the trenches with you. Let's talk honestly about how hard this might be.

Why Might This Be Hard?

Prior to having a sick child, we would have easily dismissed many of the horror stories that abound with living with an infant with acid reflux. Now that we have a child diagnosed with it (and still suffering from it) we don't dismiss a single story. In fact, we tend to think that most of those stories grossly underestimate the toll that is taken on the child's, parents', and family's quality of life.

We as humans are not hardwired to watch a child, especially an infant, be in pain. When we see a child suffering we are driven to respond. Our mind and body gear up to do whatever we need to do to help. An infant in pain makes a connection with our very soul. We are motivated. We are pushed. We *must* help.

When that child is our own, the response is raised to an entirely new level of intensity. Marian Sandmaier wrote a very poignant article for the *Washington Post* in which she described the intensity of the help-response:

> There comes a moment in a parent's life when you understand that raising a child is less an act of love and fortitude than something much wilder, something that sniffs the wind and bares its fangs at intruders, implacable in its drive to keep its offspring safe. You may not know you have this beast in you; you may see yourself as essentially rational and peaceable, willing to abide by the rules. Then everything changes.[1]

This drive to protect, to care for a little one who cannot speak and care for himself, can cause stress—a lot of stress. One of the reasons is because normal efforts to comfort usually don't work well with a baby with reflux who is in pain. An infant usually gives clear signals for the caregiver to attend to; however, the infant suffering from acid reflux may be giving unclear signals of distress and illness.[2] And therein lies one of the problems with having a baby with reflux or GERD.

Another problem with acid reflux is that it may go away quickly; however, it may last quite a while—and even a few weeks of caring for a baby with reflux can change you forever. Over a long time, this stress can mean trouble. In fact, it can mean *burnout.*

A parent who suffers burnout can become emotionally exhausted or non-caring, and feel like he or she is doing a terrible job. And those feelings unabated can turn into trouble. "Children with reflux do try the patience of a saint," says Beth Anderson, Executive Director of PAGER. "Almost all parents we talk to say this is the most stressful experience of their lives and an alarming number admit to fantasies of throwing the baby out the window."[3]

To caution you, as a caregiver of a child with reflux you may find that:

- your physical health may suffer,
- your finances may suffer,
- your mental health may suffer,
- your family life may suffer,
- your job may suffer, and
- your social life may suffer.

Your Physical Health May Suffer

Interestingly enough, when Benjamin became sick we were constantly worried about his health—and in turn ours suffered. We have always been pretty healthy folks (we are knocking on wood very hard as we write this) but, boy, did we get rocked. This isn't just a phenomenon limited to our family. There are several studies that investigated the effect that caring for a chronically ill child had on the caregiver's health. Some noted significant changes, and some even reported drastic changes to all family members' health.[4]

Our health really suffered and we believe that it was in large part due to sleep deprivation—it was one of the main problems we had. Now this is not the same type of sleep deprivation that goes along with having a healthy infant in the home, occasionally waking here and there. Oh, no! This is different—really different. It is sleep deprivation raised to a new level.

There were times when we were getting up every 19 minutes to tend to Benjamin. That in itself was difficult, but then when up, he was not consoled as a normal baby might be. He was up for hours screaming in pain and more often than not it woke the whole house.

Sleep deprivation can mean serious consequences. According to Richard Gelula of the National Sleep Foundation,

> People who sleep well, in general, are happier and healthier, but when sleep is poor or inadequate, people feel tired or fatigued, their social and intimate relationships suffer, work productivity is negatively affected, and they make our roads more dangerous by driving while sleepy and less alert.[5]

Besides the sleep issue, our backs paid a price. Why? Because our baby could not be put down; he had to be constantly held in an upright position just to relieve his pain and give him emotional support.

What accentuated the toll on our health was that the on-set of reflux was so slow and that the diagnosis was difficult to attain—it took us a year to get a definitive diagnosis. We cannot speak for others but when Benjamin was born, we were (as most parents are) somewhat braced to hear the news that something might be wrong. After several days, when everything seemed normal, we happily exhaled. However, after two weeks the reflux began to appear, when we had already taken for granted that our baby was healthy, and by that time our support team had left the job (assuming that all was well).

Your Finances May Suffer

Having a child with reflux can create a great financial burden. For instance, it was almost impossible for one of us to run off to work and leave our partner alone caring for both Benjamin and our other son. When we tried to work at home, there was no longer any peaceful space available. So we had to hire a lot of babysitters to help.

We also found that we needed extra help just to do the simple little things that we normally did before Benjamin: stuff like cleaning the house, going grocery shopping, or doing yard work. With a healthy baby, things go on, just at a much slower pace. With a reflux baby, everything can come to a screeching halt, and to get back on track you might need to spend money.

We also found that a lack of organization crept into our life with our high-needs baby. When our life got turned upside down this played havoc on our financial situation. For the first time in a 16-year marriage we missed mortgage and car insurance payments, and bounced checks.

And then there were the doctors' bills. Benjamin was at a doctor's appointment or a hospital practically every week of his life for the first six months. At one point, he was taking medication nine times per day. Even the small co-pays were adding up, not to mention the medicines that he was taking and the formula that cost over $60 a week.

And last, but by no means least, is the possibility of legal bills. Sometimes legal issues will occur that need addressing. While many parents with a baby who has a chronic illness won't encounter legal troubles it is a sad state of affairs today that some of you will. What is even sadder are the results of a recently released study that showed about half of all bankruptcies in the US are caused by medical hardship. We offer tips and suggestions about your finances in Chapter 7, "Money Matters."

Your Mental State May Suffer

We've got to tell you, your mental state may very well be at risk when dealing with a reflux baby. The disrupted social life, personal strain, economic uncertainty, and insecurity about the baby's health can all add up to a high level of stress.[6] And that is exactly what happened to us—we got worn down by the unremitting elevated level of stress.

Well, worn down isn't quite strong enough—more like crushed.

Testifying before Congress, Jan Burns, Assistant Director of PAGER, related her own experience about her child with reflux:

> I had successfully raised two other children and had a Master's degree in early intervention with 13 years of experience, but even a medical degree couldn't have prepared me for the sleep deprivation and the 24/7 intensive care parenting required to care for such a critically ill child.[7]

As Burns noted to Congress, caring for a baby with reflux can be extremely difficult. She personally related to us the following:

> Many parents report that the reflux medications do not always work. They also complain that it often takes many visits to the doctor to get proper diagnosis and treatment. So in addition to the medication not working, the first or fifth formula recommendation does not work and this leaves the parents at night crying along with the sick child.

That is pretty much what happened to us, and along the way many of our non-priority items were dropped, like exercising or going out to dinner, and that made the stress cycle build on itself.

Another thing that went was the yard and house upkeep. We just didn't have the time and energy to do the yard work and clean the house. And each time we came home and looked around, there was a constant reminder of how difficult things actually were, and of course that generated more stress.

Then, there was the strain of the unknown, and this came in three flavors. First, there was the pressure of not knowing what was wrong with Benjamin. Second, there was the pressure of not knowing for sure when he was going to get better. (People told us it would be over in three months, then in six months). Third, there was the pressure of not knowing exactly what to do to comfort Benjamin.

And lastly, with regard to your mental health there may be the need to grieve your child having an illness. But, there may be at least two problems here. Couples must grieve the loss of their expected "normal" child and work to accept the child they have. However, with reflux, sometimes the diagnosis is so slow in coming, that you only get partial insights into what is really taking place in your child and it may not be clear if your child will eventually be completely healthy or not. With a broken arm, you know, but with reflux, only time will tell what you may need to grieve. The second problem is that of sequence. As the authors related in a recent article in the *Journal of*

Nursing, there is often times a lot happening simultaneously:

> After a child is diagnosed with a chronic condition, the parents or other caregivers must quickly develop a working knowledge of the medical condition and treatment plan at a time when they are still dealing with the shock and grief of the initial diagnosis. The child's parents are also trying to process the realization that a new kind of parenting/caregiving will be required of them. They are now expected to take on the responsibility of managing the condition over time.[8]

The pressure and stress of caring for the chronically ill can be significant. There is more discussion about this in Chapter 9, "Taking Care of the Chronically Ill."

Your Family May Suffer

A reflux baby's suffering can significantly impact the quality of life for an entire family. It seems pretty reasonable to suggest that a crisis affecting one family member will affect all other family members.[9]

One of our saddest moments happened when we had directed our oldest son, Brook, to play on his own while we cared for the baby. He did something quite special while playing and he hurriedly came to report on his accomplishment, but we couldn't even hear him over Benjamin's screaming. This just added to our guilt and feelings of inadequacy, not only as parents to the baby, but now we were losing our confidence with our oldest as well.

Additionally, where days off from work were once filled with outings that included everyone, things were changed because one parent had to stay with Ben, so there was rarely a time when everyone was together.

Overall, we were just less excited about life—we were usually pretty good first thing in the morning, but when things were at their worst, we even awoke feeling defeated.

Your Job May Suffer

There has been some very interesting research done on the effects of stress in the workplace, and how that stress spills over to home life. One thing that was found was that the stress of work often came home with the worker, and does not stay at work.[10]

The same is true in the other direction—the stress of home rarely stays there; instead, it often travels to work. And that spillover to work can be very noticeable and very destructive.

When we were at work it was pretty noticeable that often we were just there physically, and not mentally. And sometimes, hardly even there physically.

Your Social Life May Suffer

Almost without saying, having a baby changes your so-cial life. This phenomenon becomes really apparent with a reflux baby, because going out with a reflux baby can often be too unpredictable. Things can get wild and crazy and can spiral out of control without warning.

One thing that we discovered was that it was extremely difficult to go out and leave Benjamin at home, because it was often too hard to find a sitter who could care for him. On the few times we did go out we would call only to hear an exasperated sitter on the line with a scream-ing baby in the background, and we quickly found our-selves on the way home.

Two months into this, already weary and exhausted be-yond our imaginations, we decided to give ourselves a break and go out and get a bite to eat. To do this we had to hire two babysitters: one for our oldest son, Brook, and one for Benjamin. Brook was very excited since we hired his favorite sitter to play with him. We were gone about an hour and on returning we found Benjamin hav-ing such a difficult time that both sitters were with him (probably in large part to give each other moral support) and poor Brook just ended up playing by himself the en-tire time.

Realize this: finding a sitter for a healthy child can be hard, but finding one to watch a child with reflux can be downright impossible.

And how about taking the child with you? Well, Sharmi Banik, a writer for the *Germantown Gazette,* describes an interesting aspect of a social life with an infant suffering with GERD:

> Imagine a casual trip to Lakeforest Mall with your baby, when suddenly he starts to scream, shake, turn blue and then projectile vomits on a well-dressed woman more than five feet away.[11]

As you might imagine, all of this can put a major crimp in any social life.

TOOL #4: How Hard Is It?

Following is an assessment that will help you evaluate the difficulty of your situation, and will suggest actions.

Needed: Form 4-1, pencil/pen, about fifteen minutes.

Step 1: Concentrate. Find some quiet time and then flip to the two-page assessment form.

Step 2: Complete the form. Answer each step to the best of your ability. You might want to consider having you and your partner complete this form separately, and then compare scores.

Step 3: Take a break. When completed, put the form down for a period of time (usually a day or two) and then review it.

Step 4: Score it. Take your score and compare it to the scale at the end of the form. From there, follow the recommendations, or consider taking action that may be appropriate for you based on the results.

FORM 4-1: HOW HARD IS IT?

To get an idea of how intense caring for your high-needs child is, answer the following questions by filling in the blanks with one of these responses that best describes your state of mind.

Excellent	Very Good	Good	Poor	Terrible
5pts	4pts	3pts	2pts	1pt

Score   Questions

1. _____ I feel that I am a(n) _____ influence on my family

2. _____ I am doing a(n) _____ job of caring for my baby.

3. _____ My relationship with my significant other is _____ .

4. _____ Compared to pre-baby, my house/apartment is in _____ condition.

5. _____ My relationships with my best friends are _____ compared to pre-baby.

6. _____ At the end of the day, my emotional state is _____ .

7. _____ I am doing a(n) _____ job my work.

8. _____   In the morning, I feel _____ .

9. _____   Being with my baby is _____ for me.

Total score: _____

Scoring. Now go back to each question. In the left-hand column give yourself the following points:

For each answer of	Give yourself
Excellent	5 points
Very good	4 points
Good	3 points
Poor	2 points
Terrible	1 point

Total it up. Now take your total score and compare it to the following chart. This will give you an idea of what action you might want to take. Keep in mind that the following are only recommendations based on common sense, and not specifically on medical guidance.

Recommendations

If you score is in this range	You might want to consider doing this:
40 to 45 points	Congratulate yourself! You're doing great.
30 to 39 points	Take special care of yourself and family members so that things don't get any worse.

| 20 to 29 points | Get support from family, friends, and support groups. Refer to the chapter "Stay Healthy" for suggestions. |
| 9 to 19 points | Talk to your general practitioner, a medical-illness therapist, or a psychologist to help you communicate to your child's doctor the level of your child's suffering.* |

* Because your child's doctor is only responsible for your child, he may not be the best person with whom to discuss your own stress.

References

1. Sandmaier, M. Listening for zebras. *The Washington Post*, June, 3, 2003.

2. Thoyre, S.M. Mothers' internal working models with infants with gastroesophageal reflux. *Maternal-Child Nursing Journal* 22:2 (1994): 39-48.

3. Fernandez, K. Bundle of misery. *The Washington Post.* August 27, 2002, F6.

4. Tomlinson, P.S., J. Kotchevar, and L. Swanson. Caregiver mental health and family health outcomes following a critical hospitalization of a child. *Issues in Mental Health Nursing* 16 (1995): 533.

5. Staff writer. Study: Most American adults sleep poorly. USA Today.com http://www.usatoday.com/news/health/2005-03-29-bad-sleep_x.htm. (Accessed 3/29/2005)

6. Patterson, J.M., B. Leonard, and J.C. Titus. Home care for medically fragile children: Impact on family health and well-being. *Development and Behavioral Pediatrics* 13 (1992): 4.

7. Staff writer. PAGER testifies before Congress. *Reflux Digest* 7:2 (June 2003): 1.

8. Sullivan-Bolyai, S., Knafl, K., Sadler, L., & Gilliss, C. Great expectations: A position description for parents as caregivers: Part 1. *Pediatric Nursing* 29, no. 6 (2004): 457-461.

9. Patterson, J.M., B. Leonard, and J.C. Titus. Home care for medically fragile children: Impact on family health and well-being. *Development and Behavioral Pediatrics* 13 (1992): 4.

10. Leiter, M. P., & Durup, J. M. (1996). Work, home, and in-between: A longitudinal study of spillover. Journal of Applied Behavioral Science, 31 (1), 29-47.

11. Banik, S. Childhood heartburn disease causes parent's grief. *Germantown Gazette*. May 18, 1994, A1.

CHAPTER 5

The Child Isn't Bad—
The Pain Is!

The first edition of this book went worldwide, and we received many positive responses. By far, the chapter that the majority of readers wrote to us about was this chapter. They wrote things like, "I am sitting at the computer, crying as I write this, with my husband looking over my shoulder. You were writing about us."

If you find yourself reading this book, especially reading this chapter, more than likely you are sleep deprived and your life/work schedule is in chaos. And you are probably at the end of your patience. It is okay. It is understandable. What you and are going through is really tough.

But your child is probably suffering even more.

We've talked to dozens upon dozens of adults who suffer from acid reflux. It absolutely floors us to hear the stories they relate about their pain, their discomfort, their altered and disrupted sleep patterns, and their descriptions of what the reflux episodes feel like.

For those of you who do not suffer from acid reflux, let us give you an idea of what the pain is like. Stomach acid is about the same pH level as the acid in an automobile battery. Can you imagine having that acid in your throat, in your nose, and maybe even in your ears several times a day? Can you imagine the episodes lasting five to ten minutes at a time?

A Baby's Reaction

Let's assume that your baby is having a severe reflux episode. The baby cannot talk so she has only one way to voice her pain—by crying (Figure 5-1). Well, probably not just crying, but instead, gut-wrenching screaming and howling that can go on and on for hours. The baby is communicating with you, and what she is telling you is:

"I AM IN PAIN! It is not my choice, I don't want it to happen, and there is nothing that I can do to stop it. I am a VICTIM here too!"

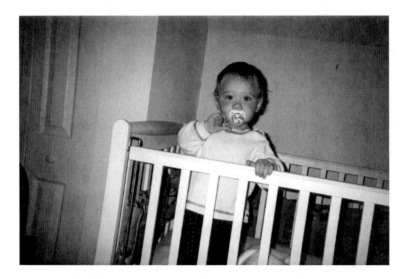

Figure 5-1. Babies don't have a voice to explain their pain.

A Child's Reaction

So much became clear to us just before our son Ben's third birthday. It was a Saturday and it had been a rough one. We decided Ben had cried and screamed more that day than his nine-year-old brother had cried his entire toddler-hood. Then, that evening, when we were walking with Ben, he looked up at us and said, "I am sorry I was bad today. My acid reflux was bothering me." That was huge for us for two reasons.

First, we finally had some solid indication that his behavior was somewhat explained by his discomfort from reflux. Secondly, we saw that point in time as a family milestone. After so many days and nights of crying, he was finally beginning to be able put words to his pain.

Acid Reflux in Infants and Children

There doesn't seem to be consensus on how children react to pain. Where one toddler may scream in pain, another may grow silent, or distant. Where one child with reflux may want to drink constantly to help correct the problem, another may begin to abandon food because it hurts. You just don't know, and that's just one of your challenges. Here are two examples of different reactions submitted by readers of this book's first edition:

> Justin had a hard time sleeping and had a difficult time being on his stomach. He also made a swallowing sound and gesture after feedings. It was as if his milk kept coming up his throat and he kept pushing it down by swallowing. He cried and screamed most of the time in those moments. It seemed to get worse in the afternoons.
>
> — Valery F.
> Quebec, Canada

> Clayton does not eat well and sleeps very poorly. He wakes two or more times per night, sometimes for an hour or more. He screams and is inconsolable. He gets rigid, throws back his head, arching his neck. Food aversion and refusals are the norm at this time and all he wants to do is drink.
>
> — Jacquelyn N.
> New Jersey

A Parent's Reaction

Parents of a healthy baby are usually asked to tend to a crying baby every so often. For them, it is easy to respond with infinite patience, caring words, and great empathy. However, parents of a baby with reflux are asked to respond to a baby in discomfort almost continuously. Additionally, common methods of comforting the baby usually don't work, and this can be more than discouraging. Another challenge is that the signals you receive from a child suffering from reflux may be unclear signals of distress and illness. Because of all this and more, it is sometimes difficult to remember it is not the baby that is bad, but it is the baby's pain that is bad.

It is therefore important that you respond appropriately to the only language the baby or child has. One way to check in to see if you are is by reviewing the language that you use to describe your child's situation. For instance, saying that your baby is "fussy," "precocious," or "demanding" suggests that you think that your baby might be making a conscious decision to be in pain or to frequently wake up. That is pretty darn unlikely.

To help determine if you responding as well as you can, go to Tool #5, "Are You Blaming the Child?"

A Physician's Reaction

We are sorry to report that in the search to get our son better, we had to "kiss a lot of frogs" who were posing as knowledgeable health-care providers. When Benjamin's symptoms first appeared we were told everything under the sun to explain his intense crying—from it was the "mom's fault," to he was "precocious," to he was just "trying to get attention." It became apparent that either we were not explaining his symptoms well enough or his pain was not being taken seriously.

We also found some amazing health-care providers, who were more like "princes and princesses." You will find some of their words of wisdom in this book.

We found that how each physician responded to reflux seemed to be as varied as how each child and adult responds to reflux. However, we found that the more experienced, knowledgeable, and up-to-date on the research related to reflux that the health-care provider was, the more empathetic and direct was his or her response to our child's pain.

Fortunately for those following behind us, it appears that there will soon be more "kings and queens" out there to choose from. One reason is that the under-treatment of pain is now being taken more seriously, by more than just parents. In fact, recognizing that under-treatment of pain is a public health priority, the Federation of State Medical Boards of the United States, Inc., is recommending a revision of guidelines stating that under-treatment of pain, like over-treatment, is a practice violation.[1]

Pain related to reflux is also being more closely considered. New research is shedding light on the connections between reflux, damage, and pain. It now appears that a person can still have severe reflux without having damage to the esophagus. In fact, one researcher noted that up to 75 percent of people with acid reflux do not have erosion of the lining of the esophagus.[2] What this means is that a baby or child may not present with signs of physical damage to the esophagus but could still be suffering significant pain. And we know from our own experience with our son that it does not always take a very low pH level to generate pain, especially if the reflux travels into the upper esophagus.

If a physician is not experienced with reflux then he or she may become impatient when there is not a quick fix. Unfortunately, this can lead to frustration and blame. This happens more than it should with infant reflux. Here is one such story related in *Reflux Digest*:

> Our son . . . suffered with reflux from birth. He was 15 months of age before I found anyone who would really believe just how much pain he almost constantly endured. He woke crying in very real pain anywhere from 8 to 14 times each and every night.[3]

TOOL #5: Are You Blaming the Child?

The following examples may give some insight into the importance of your communication.

Step 1: Your words are important. A vital step in not blaming the baby/child for the pain is using words that describe the child's innocence. Your words are incredibly powerful and often set the tone for your mood and your ability to care for your baby.

Step 2: Listen. Register in your mind which of the following examples of communication do and do not blame the child for being in pain.

Blaming the Child	Blaming the Pain
The child kept me up all night last night.	The child had a difficult night last night.
The child wouldn't let me put him down all day.	He really needed me to hold him all day to provide him some relief.
The child just spit up on my new sweater and ruined it.	The child wasn't able to keep his food down.
The child's constant crying is driving me nuts.	The child seems especially uncomfortable today.

Step 3: Notice any trends? Now listen to your own references to your child's and family's discomfort and try to be conscious of how you are expressing the situation. Notice any similarities to the choices above?

Your words, your language, can give you insight into how you view your child's pain, and this is critical. We found that once we could get our arms around the pure agony that Benjamin was going through we were much better able to help him, and in turn improve the quality of his and our lives (Figure 5-2).

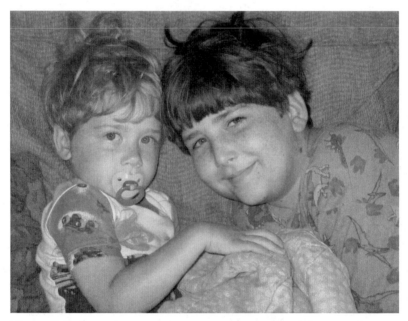

Figure 5-2. As we began to better manage Benjamin's pain, his older brother began to really enjoy having a little brother.

References
    1. Barclay L. Revised pain management guidelines target inadequate pain control: a newsmaker interview with James N. Thompson, MD. Medscape Medical News. Available at: http://www.medscape.com/viewarticle/472893. (Accessed: April 4, 2004.)

2. Pallarito, K. GERD: It's more than just heartburn. *Health-Day News.* November 23, 2004.

3. Letter to the editor. *Reflux Digest* 5:2 (Summer 2001): 10.

CHAPTER 6

Taking Care of Yourself

L ike many Americans, we have been blessed with relatively good health. Besides the occasional bout with the flu, colds, and the assorted sports-related injuries, our lives have been pretty healthy. That is until Ben's illness.

Within the last three years, Mike had bronchitis several times and numerous sinus infections, our oldest son had croup multiple times, and Tracy had a spell of blurred vision that lasted for what seemed an eternity.

At the onset of Ben's illness, we became greatly focused on caring for him and in turn our own health began to pay the price. This became very evident after one hospital stay in the spring of 2003. After two days of testing and wonderful care at Georgetown University Hospital, the three of us (Tracy, Benjamin, and Mike) came home. By the time we got back, both adults became very sick with strep throat. Now strep throat in itself is not exactly a pleasant experience but what made it worse was that we were so run down that even with treatment of antibiotics we could not shake it. It took several return visits to the doctors' offices and long courses of medication to finally recover. We believe that our immune systems had become so drained from lack of sleep that we became more susceptible to illness.

Research is now emerging that explains the seriousness of the lack of sleep related to acid reflux. The first major multi-center, randomized, double-blind, placebo-controlled trial addressing therapy for gastroesophageal reflux disease–related sleep disorders was published in the September 2005 issue of the *American Journal of Gastroenterology*. This research indicated that there is an enormous price being paid for lack-of-sleep problems related to reflux.[1] The study revealed that U.S. workers who frequently suffer from moderate-to-severe nighttime heartburn symptoms cost the U.S. economy $1.9 billion per week in paid hours of lost productivity. "Sleep problems are extremely common in patients with GERD and are often unrecognized," said lead author David A. Johnson, M.D.

That estimate was for workers who themselves suffered from GERD. However, a little common sense suggests that when a child suffers sleep problems from GERD the parents or caregivers will also suffer sleep problems.

It is estimated that an adult needs, on average, seven to eight hours of sleep a night. Yet, when caring for a child suffering from acid reflux, that amount of sleep may be reduced to as little as three to five hours per night. Over a period of time, that lack of sleep adds up.

And there are two other statistics that suggest to us that lack of sleep can be of greater importance than just a money issue. First, in 2004 there were over 100,000 motor vehicle accidents caused by drivers falling asleep at the wheel. Second, those accidents contributed to 1500 deaths.

And while we do not want to overwhelm you with news about a reality that you may already be experiencing, we want to convince you of the seriousness of the situation if you find yourself in the position of caring for a chronically ill baby or child. Recent research in this area is also indicating that the effects can be lasting.

In a recent article in *Web MD Medical News,* scientists looked at how chronic stress may lead to premature aging.[2] The study looked at 58 healthy women, all mothers of either a healthy child or a chronically ill child. The results suggested that the cells from highly-stressed mothers (taking care of a chronically-ill child) had aged from 9 to 17 years compared with the cells from the low-stressed mothers (caring for a healthy child).

We keep in mind these words that someone wise imparted to us: "The healthier you are, the better care you can give to your child." Caregiving for the chronically ill can take a toll. That is why you should take steps to insure your own health. Following are two steps we consider critical to helping you do just that.

Step 1: Recharge Your Own Batteries

Back in the early 1970s, the United States went through a pretty tough time called the Energy Crisis. As a country we were consuming more energy than we produced so we had to import it. The folks we were importing it from decided they weren't going to give us any more and whammo, we had a crisis. Well, if you are not careful as a caregiver of a child with acid reflux, you may well suffer your own energy crisis.

Many of us like to think that we can run on and on like the Energizer Bunny^{TM}. However, as we just discussed, that's not so, and your batteries will run down. (Notice the choice of word: *will* instead of *might*.)

To keep it simple, we like to describe recharging your batteries as finding your emotional, physical, or spiritual center; nourishing your soul; or practicing self-care to maintain your emotional health.

We know from experience that maintaining your emotional health is typically low on the list of daily priorities when you are taking care of a child with acid reflux. So the challenge in recharging your batteries is to search for sources of renewal in your daily routines. (Unless you know something we don't, that exotic Caribbean vacation probably isn't happening anytime soon. To show you what we mean, we both haven't been to a dinner and a movie alone since the turn of the century.)

In our case, many well-meaning friends, relatives, and caregivers tried early on to suggest breaks for us that just weren't realistic. Unless you had spent time with Ben, you had no idea how hard it was to leave him alone. For instance, when Tracy took Ben to visit her mom in Florida, her mother told her, "Go take a break and have some fun." When Tracy returned after only a few hours, Tracy's mom was sitting on her bed, with a screaming baby and said, "It scares me how hard Ben is crying. I don't think I will be able to do that again!" (She has since helped in so many other ways, as grandmothers always do.)

So, to keep it realistic, recharging your own batteries may be as simple as...

- Positive self-talk ("We can do this, we can do this...")

- Reading a chapter from a favorite book (notice we had the experience not to suggest the whole book?)

- Taking a bath and lighting a candle (with earplugs)

- Taking a few minutes for prayer or meditation

- Having a focused conversation (or e-mail) with a friend

- Attending one support group meeting (moms' or dads' group or reflux- or feeding-support group, for example)

- Doing any amount of exercise that you can sneak in

- Learning something new (Tracy has learned to roller blade 15 minutes at a time since Benjamin's birth)

Those are some of the recharging activities that we do. Yours may be totally different. The point is to begin to incorporate something into your daily routine.

Step 2: Call in the Cavalry

Little doubt about it, our first year with Benjamin was one of the hardest physical and mental things we had ever done. We had both participated in competitive collegiate sports and this was much tougher. There is no way that we could have done it without support—a lot of support—from our family, friends, and acquaintances.

When we first became aware of Benjamin's illness we were hesitant to ask for help outside of the medical profession. This was for a couple of reasons. One, for example, was our sense of pride—we felt like we should be able to handle this, especially when we were often told that it was just a "little bit" of reflux. Another reason was that we didn't have a clue how bad his illness was and the effect it would have on us. And yet another was that we didn't want to burden people with our problems. However, six months into the process, our physical and mental condition dictated to us to ask for help.

You see, life before a new baby is a lot like driving a brand new car down the road on a nice, straight highway. You can pretty much go where you want, when you want. However, when you add a new healthy baby to your family you can still keep on driving, although for a while it's going to be difficult to keep going without some stops here and there. However, when you have a baby with acid reflux it is like someone is constantly putting the parking brake on. You go nowhere, and nowhere fast. And that was actually our family's code name for a really bad day with Ben; we would say that we had been "braked!"

When Ben's illness was at its worst, our yard was a mess, the garden looked like a bomb had gone off in it, and it seemed like an F3 tornado had touched down inside our house. Our cars were hanging on by a thread and we missed bill deadlines left and right. We looked and felt terrible and were grossly sleep deprived. Our two small businesses were greatly affected. Our number one son was definitely playing second fiddle as we spent most of our time caring for Ben. And our jobs . . . well, let's just say that we were very lucky to have understanding bosses and seniority at both of our jobs. And lucky to keep our jobs.

Life had gone to hell in a handbasket and it became apparent that it was time to call in the cavalry. The first to respond were our families, second our friends, and third our co-workers. In short time we had frequent dinners being made for us, folks helping with our eldest son, people spending the night once a week so we could sleep, and people helping out in more ways than we could ever imagine. The difference it made was very significant.

However, before you sound the alarm and call in the support troops, let us impart this word of warning based on our experiences. We found that the people who had a history with us and who cared about us were the ones who responded quickly and caringly. Be cautious about reaching out to people with whom you don't have a relationship. These people, especially if they have never had a sick child, may misinterpret you or your request for help.

All right, with that out in the open, here are some people and places that you may consider reaching out to:

Your partner. As simple as this might sound, the first place you should look for support is in your partner. In our case we both worked on Ben's care equally. However, in some relationships this doesn't happen for a variety of reasons (e.g., job constraints).

Friends. If you decide to approach your friends you will probably be as surprised at their reactions as we were. We found some friends who we assumed were going to be helpful and supportive but who weren't and just disappeared. For them, it was beyond their capacity to help. At the other end of the spectrum were friends who were so supportive that it blew us away; and we even found some friends whose children had had similar problems when they were babies (those were the folks who were always holding Benjamin while we ate).

In Chapter 9, Dr. Wirtz mentions the importance of dialogue with others, especially those who may be dealing with similar challenges. We can voice support for his opinion from our own experience because we have found several other families who are dealing with their own chronic, taxing situations and with whom we communicate frequently. One family is dealing with cancer, another family has had a parent stationed away from home at the Pentagon since 9/11, and the third family is dealing with a high-needs foster child. In fact, we jokingly call ourselves the "dysfunctionals," and find the group of friends a safe place to tell stories about how atypical some days seem to be. (The joke is, after someone unleashes a story about how difficult a day was, someone in the background is always there to yell out, "Give me a 'D'!") We even have some simple rules for our almost weekly gatherings. We have the children join us because it is often too difficult or expensive to find babysitters. No one is allowed to do any house cleaning for the get-togethers (we make a point of inspecting the host family's floor for any vacuum tracks), and we don't make fancy food the focus. Everyone brings something, and often it is as simple as gathering in the park for peanut butter and jelly sandwiches and a bag of chips. The most important point of the gathering is to support each other. Period.

Your workplace. Make full use of your sick leave. To help that happen you may want to make sure your supervisor understands exactly what you are going through (this may require medical documentation). Also, you may find your coworkers more sympathetic than you can imagine, since many adults suffer from acid reflux.

Family. You may or may not have family members in a position to help. Not everyone is lucky enough to have an aunt next door, as in days gone by, or a grandfather who can dedicate an afternoon (Figure 6-1). However, even family members far away can help. For example, Tracy's sister has a very demanding job so is not able to help out much in person but has helped financially with some of the extra expenses related to Ben's health care. Her brother also has a demanding job but has a weekend house nearby where we can hide away at times to take a nap or have a much needed uninterrupted conversation.

Support groups. There are support groups for just about any situation you can imagine. For children with GER and GERD there are several. A list can be found in the resource section of this book.

Babysitters. It used to be that you hired a babysitter and then vacated the premises—went out to dinner or a movie. We found that we had to hire a babysitter just so we could pick up around the house or spend time with our other child. Most of our hours writing this book have been at home, with a babysitter. Ben can still be a pretty high-maintenance guy and counting on an uninterrupted hour or two is just not reasonable at this point without a little outside assistance.

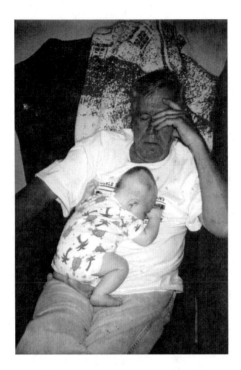

Figure 6-1. A part of our cavalry, Grandfather rests after a long day.

Church. Most churches have some type of a caring committee for families in need. If you belong to a church, be sure to let the appropriate people at your church know what is happening. There may also be financial assistance available from your church to help with some of the medical expenses. One of the Elders in our church informed us about a trust that was available to help families in difficult situations, and we were able to write a grant to help with some of our expenses.

Your own doctor. Often if your child has severe reflux or GERD, you will be seeing a specialist such as a gastroenterologist. Keep in contact with your own personal doctor. Make an appointment and inform him or her exactly what is happening in your life. Explain that you have concerns about your own health in this situation.

The physician may be able to make suggestions for your health and he or she may have resources for your family. In Mike's case, his general practitioner had gone through a similar experience with his own child so he was very sensitive to what Mike was experiencing. In fact, often when Mike went to the doctor, a significant amount of time was spent talking about Benjamin and what to do to help.

A mental health professional. The stress and strain of taking care of a child with reflux can be incredibly intense. A psychologist or other mental health professional can help you organize your thoughts related to the care of your child and keep you on track with your own self care. (Besides, if your insurance pays for it, think of it as an hour of much needed "quiet" time!).

Following are two useful tools to help you take care of yourself.

TOOL #6: Do You Need Support?

This exercise can serve two purposes. Not only does it help you see possible areas in your life that may need more attention, but it can also lead you in a conversation with family members about what is, or isn't, a priority in your life right now while you have a high-needs baby or child.

Sometimes it helps just to have such a conversation with your partner about what is important now and what is not. Such discussions can give each other permission to let go of some of the stress, or it can let your partner and/or family know the areas that really mean a lot to you, and those areas can become more of a focus.

Step 1: Do you need the cavalry? If you have a child with acid reflux, how complicated the reflux is will determine if you need support in other areas of your life. For example, Benjamin's case was (and still is) complex, and as noted in this chapter, we needed a lot of help.

To determine if you might need more support than you already have, we have included a simple chart. You will find multiple areas that tend to get neglected when intensive childcare is required. To use the chart, circle the appropriate number that represents the current condition of an area as compared to how it was before your baby with reflux. (Feel free to put other areas in; the ones listed were affected the greatest in our life.)

Chart 6-1. HOW ARE THINGS?

1) How does the interior of your house look now, compared to before you had a baby with acid reflux?

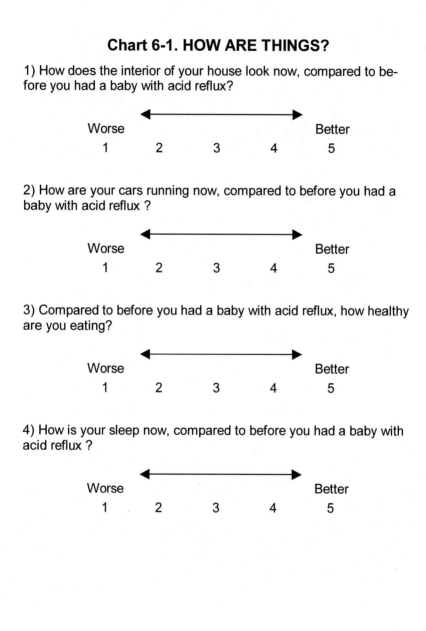

2) How are your cars running now, compared to before you had a baby with acid reflux ?

3) Compared to before you had a baby with acid reflux, how healthy are you eating?

4) How is your sleep now, compared to before you had a baby with acid reflux ?

5) How does your yard look now, compared to before you had a baby with acid reflux?

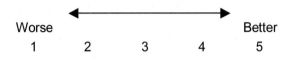

Worse   Better

1   2   3   4   5

6) How are you doing paying your bills compared to before you had a baby with acid reflux?

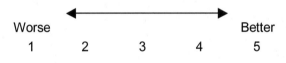

Worse   Better

1   2   3   4   5

7) How is your attention to your other child(ren) now, compared to before you had a baby with acid reflux?

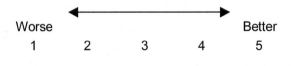

Worse   Better

1   2   3   4   5

8) How is the quality of time you are spending with your partner now, compared to before you had a baby with acid reflux?

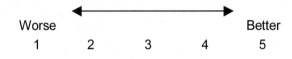

Worse   Better

1   2   3   4   5

9) How is your stress level now, compared to before you had a baby with acid reflux?

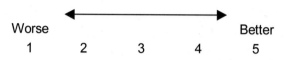

Worse				Better
1	2	3	4	5

10) How is your job performance now, compared to before you had a baby with acid reflux?

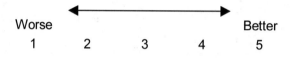

Worse				Better
1	2	3	4	5

Determine your score. Add up the numbers that you have circled. Your total is: _____ .

In general, how are you doing? Now take your total and compare it to the following:

If your point total is:	You should:
10 to 20	Get support, and fast.
21 to 30	Work on getting support as soon as you can.
31 to 50	Pat yourself on the back because you are doing great.

TOOL #7: Recharging Your Batteries

Answer the following questions for valuable insights into ways that you might recharge your batteries.

1) How do you care for yourself each day?

2) What activities give you renewed energy?

3) What activities calm you?

4) If you had just 15 minutes each day, what could you add to your routine to renew your spirit?

5) Pre-kid(s), what did you do to relax? Can you do something similar?

6) Make a list of quickie relaxers and put them in a conspicuous place for all to see.

References

1. Johnson, D. Effect of esomeprazole on nighttime heartburn and sleep quality in patients with GERD: A randomized, placebo-controlled trial. *American Journal of Gastroenterology* 100, no. 9 (2005): 1914-22.

2. Davis, J. Chronic stress may make cells age faster. *WebMD News*. (Nov. 29, 2004). <http://www.webmd.com/content/-article/97/104269.htm> (Accessed Jul 2005).

CHAPTER 7

Money Matters

This may blow over very quickly—two months from now, this could all be a distant memory. In fact, you may not even have time to get to the bank, and it's over. After all, a majority of kids outgrow reflux before their first birthday.

However, as we write this book, Ben is three and a half years old and still has reflux, and the financial burdens continue to be great. We are writing this to tell you that there may be a chance, even if your child has reflux for a short period of time, that you may spend a lot of money (even if you have good health insurance) to care for your child.

Although the full range of costs associated with pediatric reflux has not been studied, nor have the costs associated with lack of treatment,[1] in a study released in February 2005, Harvard University researchers offered a pair of startling findings: First, half of all bankruptcies in the U.S. stem from a medical crisis—and the group hardest hit was the middle class. Second, of the 700,000 households that are driven into bankruptcy each year by medical crisis, three-quarters had health insurance at the onset of their illness, more than half were homeowners, and 50 percent included a member with a college education.[2]

Expenses

Here are just a few of the related expenses you might run into if your child has reflux (not necessarily in order of priority):

Medication(s). There are a variety of medications that reflux children are often treated with. (One of our friend's daughters who had reflux was taking 12 medications at the age of 6.)

Formula(s). Oftentimes formulas are changed in an attempt to find one that helps reduce the reflux symptoms. Some formulas can be very expensive and are seldom covered by health insurance.

Doctor and hospital visits. Reflux is recognized as a chronic condition, which means that you may be seeing a lot of doctors, and that can be expensive—even a simple co-pay can begin to add up. If the reflux is very severe, surgery, and all of the associated expenses, may be necessary.

Babysitters. If you have other young children, it is inevitable that you will need to enlist the help of others to care for them.

Dry cleaning and laundry. If you've got a refluxer who vomits you'll probably be doing a lot of laundry—a whole lot.

Special care items. Babies with reflux often need to sleep on an incline, and to be carried in an upright position. Chances are that you'll need unique items such as a crib that can incline, special carriers, or even a sling-type device to keep the infant positioned appropriately when sleeping.

Legal bills. There is a chance, a slim one, albeit still a chance, that you might need to engage the services of a lawyer.

To help you get a picture of the possible cost associated with a baby with reflux, we thought it might be helpful to highlight some of our expenses associated with Ben's illness during his first year of life.

Ben had over 50 doctor visits ($10 co-pay each) and five different hospital admissions in four different hospitals (one was at the University of Missouri, which meant that we had to fly our other child to his grandmother's in Florida [$500]). He took seven medications for his reflux (approximately $10 each week) and was on a special formula ($60 a week). Due to the misfortune of spending too much time early on with doctors who didn't know much about reflux, we had incurred some legal bills.

Of course this accounting did not include missed work, or the cost of the extra help we needed to have around the house, or the special groceries we bought at the health food store because his stomach was so sensitive.

Our purpose in sharing this is not to scare you, but we wish that we would have known ahead of time what the fiscal implications of this "Oh-don't-worry-he'll-outgrow-it-in-a-few-months-just-a-little-bit-of-reflux-looks-fine-to-me-seems-to-be-thriving" disease were. As the Harvard study showed, a chronic illness can have a major financial impact on all kinds of families, even the middle class with good health insurance. For the past three years, our out-of-pocket medical expenses related to Ben's reflux have been more than $12,000 each year.

TOOL #8: Assessing Your Financial Situation

The following exercise can help you determine if there may be a financial disaster looming on your horizon.

As much as some people would like you to believe differently, no one can predict the future, especially when it comes to your finances. However, with a little groundwork, you can get a pretty accurate idea of your current situation and an indication of what the future may bring.

There is one thing that we know with absolute certainty. When you have a chronically ill child, your financial situation will change.

Step 1: Seek help. With that thought hanging out there—that your situation will change—one of the best things that you can do for yourself is to seek out the guidance of a financial advisor.

Okay, so you might have a fancy program on your computer that tracks all your money, or a hefty rainy-day fund. So did we, and we got financially rocked. Between the medications, doctor appointments, travel, formulas, and so on, the rainy-day fund quickly evaporated and we found ourselves really struggling with money. One of our saving graces was our accountant. He looked at our finances from an objective perspective and made recommendations that made all the difference in the world.

Step 2: Who are you looking for? We suggest that you seek someone who can perform a current account of your finances. This might be an accountant or a financial advisor. Or it might be a friend. Regardless of the title of the person, there are two traits you are looking for. One is trust. Can you and do you trust the person? That is paramount. The other is the person's knowledge. Does he or she know what is necessary to help?

Step 3: What are you looking for? Simply, you are looking for two things. One is the bottom line on personal worth. In particular, what is your worth at this point in time, and what resources do you have available (e.g., cash, equity) if you were to need them? The second is your current money flow. Are you spending more money than you have coming in? Those two items can give you an idea of what your flow is.

Why do you want to know this? Of course, you want to avoid financial disaster. However, you also want to keep your money situation from adding to the stress that you and your family are already experiencing.

Step 4: It's a positive. If the determination is that your flow is positive (income is greater than expenses), great. Keep paying the bills and build up a rainy day fund as much as possible. Financially speaking, what we found with Benjamin was that there were some sunny days; however, there were a lot of rainy days, and there were a few hurricane days with more rain than we had ever imagined.

Step 5: It's a wash. If your flow turns out to be zero (income equals expenses) trouble might be just ahead. The main reason is that it doesn't give you much wiggle room in case your money requirements change. So we suggest that you scrimp and save as much as possible and build up a cushion. Why? With reflux, especially severe reflux, complications can occur that need treatment that can be expensive. For instance, Benjamin picked up a stomach virus that in combination with his reflux was terrible. That put him in the hospital for six days.

Step 6: It's a negative. If your flow is negative (income is less than expenses), trouble is here. Sooner or later, probably sooner, there will be a reckoning. At this point we cannot recommend strongly enough to get assistance and develop a plan.

Don't turn a blind eye to this. Even if you're an optimist, if your child has reflux, you've got enough stress in your life. You don't need money issues to compound that stress. So to keep the stress from building, we suggest that you take positive steps as soon as you can, and get someone, and it may be the person who helped you determine your flow, to help you with a plan.

We had to do this, and our accountant presented several things that needed to be done. We had to make some very difficult choices, but those choices made an enormous difference in our stress level, helping us avoid financial disaster.

Two of those choices involved our respective retirement plans. We decided that one of us would make early withdraws from the account, while the other would stop making contributions. Both steps increased our available cash and really made a difference.

Here are a few other things you might consider doing: ask doctors for samples of medications, work with your insurance company to pay for special formulas, look for rebates on medications, and check with local civic organizations to help with you with a specific large ticket item like a far-away hospital visit.

References

1. Staff writer. PAGER testifies before Congress. *Reflux Digest* 7:2 (June 2003): 4.

2. Smolowe, J., L. Gray, A. Driscoll, C. Love, S. Schrobsdorff, and R. Schlesinger. Destroyed by doctor bills. *People* (February 14, 2005): 105-8.

PART 3

Discussions from Experts in the Field

Many experts have made significant contributions to Benjamin's care. The following exceptional health-care professionals have graciously donated their time to share their expertise and wisdom with you. Be fore-warned, the following chapters will get progressively more technical and detailed.

♦ Patients without Words

♦ Caring for the Chronically Ill

♦ Nutrition for the Child with Acid Reflux

♦ Food Allergy and Reflux

♦ Extra-Esophageal Reflux and Symptoms of the Ear, Nose, and Throat

♦ The Use of Medications in Acid-Reflux Disease

CHAPTER 8

Patients Without Words

Kim Fincher, DVM

M edicine is said to be half science and half art. The science part can be frustrating in that there are few "hard and fast," easy diagnoses and few "black and whites," but many shades of gray. And nowhere is the "art" half of the equation so important as in the patient without words.

Animals, infants, and some geriatric patients share an obstacle to diagnosis and treatment of their medical conditions in that they cannot describe them. This is not an insurmountable problem as long as two basic requirements exist. First, their caretakers must be astute observers and recorders of everyday signs and symptoms. Secondly, health-care professionals must carefully digest and analyze these data frequently in order to manage and to (ultimately) cure difficult cases.

Veterinarians never have the luxury of patients who can describe their own symptoms. We therefore rely completely upon our own physical examinations, daily observations by the caregiver, diagnostic tests, and response to treatment by our patients. In school we are taught to "look at the patient" as a reminder that clinical signs cannot be ignored in our efforts to gather sophisticated data and to manage complex cases.

Where to Start

As a parent of a child with a chronic condition, you must know that, by definition, "chronic" means not solved simply. The encouraging news is that there is help for both you and your child through diligence and persistence. Despite sleep deprivation, fatigue, and all of your work and home distractions, you are the best advocate for your child because you are with him/her 24/7. All of the symptoms, drug successes and failures, side effects, sleep patterns, nutrition and behaviors will be observed by you. No physician, no matter how specialized or brilliant, can visit with your child (even repeatedly) and solve the mystery of his individual problems without you.

Observe and record. Many of your observations may seem meaningless at first, but if simple notes are recorded with a date and time, some patterns and correlations can be discovered. Parents in a sleep-deprived state may not be able to recall which night their child awakened every hour or what he had eaten before the six-hour uninterrupted sleep. Write notes frequently to prepare for the day that a physician will begin to diagnose and treat your child.

Find help. There are many health professionals in many different fields whom you may need along the way. Their most important qualification may be that they can listen to you, the caregiver. When setting up appointments, communicate clearly to the receptionist that you have many concerns or problems. Ask for a day or time when the physician is best able to address them, acknowledging extra cost to you if an extended visit is required. Be selective. Any member of the team who is unable or unwilling to listen to your questions and help you find answers can be replaced.

Know what to expect. Because you are reading this book, you have already determined that there are no simple solutions to your child's problems. Remind yourself that many small steps are required to reach every distant goal. Diagnosis and treatment always begin with a lengthy history (taken from all of those observations) and physical exam, sometimes by several different professionals. Your child will then need a battery of basic tests to establish his baseline data. Specialized tests, though, are often done best by specialists.

Before submitting to invasive procedures, ask how often the person has performed them and what can be gained with the results. Be prepared to travel to experts where similar patients are seen frequently rather than staying local and getting inclusive results. (Some physicians have other patients' permission to be called as references.) All patients without words deserve the special attention that is required to maximize their quality of life. And no one is better equipped to speak for a child than you, the caregiver.

Reaching a Diagnosis and Treatment Plan

Diagnosis. Careful analysis of your observations over time and a set of standard and specialized tests should lead to a list of differential diagnoses. (Remember that response to treatment can be diagnostic in itself. For example, a fever that responds to an antibiotic is bacterial rather than viral.) Don't forget to look at the patient. If tests results are all normal, but your child is not well (underweight, not sleeping, regurgitating frequently, showing no improvement over time), keep looking. More tests may be required or a different treatment tried. Perhaps your regular physician is as frustrated as you are and would like to refer you elsewhere.

Treatment plan. Once a diagnosis is confirmed, a treatment plan should follow. This may include changes in daily care (thickened formula feedings in smaller volumes, sleeping on an incline, etc.) and/or pharmaceuticals. The obvious basic questions then are: What is a reasonable goal of treatment and how long should it take (the best-case scenario); what are possible side effects and toxicities (the worst-case scenario); and when might we need to adjust the plan? These are difficult questions that may require a visit with your physician without your child present to distract you or them. A follow-up visit or phone consultation should be scheduled to answer questions and concerns that arise early in the treatment process.

Advocacy. Parents, caregivers and physicians all advocate for the patient without words in their own way. In the case of a chronically ill or difficult-to-diagnose child, all of you deserve praise for meeting the challenge to maximize the patient's quality of life. Parents, caregivers, and physicians all advocate by questioning and keeping appointments, by observing and doing research, by enduring tests and giving treatments, and by not giving up. Good health care is only possible through good communication and perseverance by all of the patient's advocates.

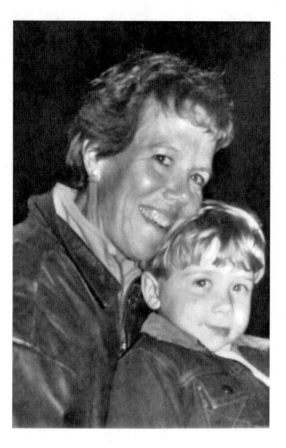

Author Dr. Kim Fincher with Ben.

CHAPTER 9

Caring for the Chronically Ill

Richard Wirtz, PsyD

As a young, energetic college kid trying to earn some money during the summer I unloaded boxcars at a warehouse. I'd be working right from the start of the day, sun beating down on that steel boxcar, temperature and humidity in the 90s and the old guys they brought in for temporary help would be shaking their heads.

One day the oldest and strongest guy who always seemed to get the assignment to come to the warehouse said, "Son, you gotta pace yourself. You got all day to unload this car." It probably took me 20 more years to grasp the wisdom of that advice—not about boxcars, but about approaching a physically and mentally draining task.

It is in this sense that managing a chronic illness is about pacing yourself. It's about being aware that you are running a marathon, not a sprint, and that doing so successfully requires a very different set of strategies.

It's All about the Pace

Now, for the experienced marathoners reading this chapter it will be all too apparent that I've never run one, at least not one of the 26-mile variety, so humor me a little as I oversimplify the process to make a point. A marathon is about endurance. It is not some blinding burst of speed that only needs to be sustained for a matter of seconds. It is a taxing, persistent effort over a long and sometimes very challenging course.

In order to succeed at managing a chronic illness, you must find the pace or rhythm that you can sustain in your day-to-day life with a chronically ill child or family member. This means identifying a realistic set of expectations and activities that match the realities of your unique situation. For example, if your child only sleeps four hours a night (which means you sleep less!), working a full-time job; being super parent, spouse, homeowner, lover, socialite, and church member; and leaping over tall buildings in a single bound are not all going to be possible.

So you pare down to bare necessities whenever possible—like those skimpy little shorts that the marathoners wear—just the necessities! This leaves room for other people to be superheroes. This idea is very hard for many folks because they have lots of "I should…" and "I ought to be able to …" messages in their heads, which are deeply held ideas about how you are supposed to be able to do things and what you are supposed to be able to accomplish.

This is sometimes complicated by the ignorance of others around you who do not fully understand what this experience is like. Their lack of understanding may be a product of having been spared the gory details or simply not being able to *really* grasp what this experience is like. Lucky them! However, sometimes you may have to enlighten them so that they can respond more appropriately when you've "hit the wall," or in order to help *prevent* you from doing so.

Staying Focused on <u>Now</u>

Another important concept in successful marathoning is never looking or thinking too far ahead. The idea of having 20 more miles to go can really ruin a good endorphin buzz and takes your focus off what you need to do next. At the risk of throwing too many clichés in here, the Alcoholic Anonymous saying "One day at a time" is particularly pertinent.

Identifying what you need to do for your child or yourself at this particular moment, during the next hour, or for the rest of the day puts the task in a much more manageable perspective. Just as the runner focuses on her form as she takes the next stride, you can be most effective when you stay focused on the task at hand, in the moment.

Obviously, there is a need for strategy, and that requires brief shifts of focus to what's coming up next, for example: picking up your child at the bus stop on time, getting to the pharmacy before it closes, not missing the doctor's appointment that you've been waiting three weeks for, and other important jobs. But just as the runner tries to envision the next stretch of the course to make decisions about pace, positioning in the pack, or making a move on the runner ahead, she has to come back to focus on form, handling the exchange of the water cup, and so on, to be able to accomplish those goals. Asking yourself what you need right now, this instant, or what your child must have right now, in this moment, will help you manage what the next hour, day, week, month, or year has in store.

Taking Care of Yourself

If you are like most parents who care enough about their children to read a book like this, you are likely to be much better at identifying your child's needs than your own. That seems like the right order of priorities in the beginning when there are so many unanswered questions and frightening experiences. However, as the condition clearly evolves from acute to chronic there *must* be a shift in the balance to something that more closely resembles even. There is no way around it: if you do not take care of yourself, you will be unable to respond to anything but the most acute situations.

While being able to respond to a crisis is important, it no longer characterizes the bulk of your experiences and therefore many opportunities to really "be with" your child will be lost. So, how much sleep do you typically get? What have your eating habits been like lately? When was the last time you exercised, other than when you lug laundry up from the basement? What was the last movie you saw? (They've come out with some pretty good ones since *Star Wars*!) Has it occurred to you that watching *Friends* reruns does not qualify as a social life? And then there is sexual intimacy with your partner.... Are you seeing a pattern here?

Asking for Help

The issue of taking care of yourself, which is so critical to being able to care for your child, brings us to another major hurdle for some folks: *asking for and/or accepting help.* Wouldn't running the marathon be so much more manageable if you only had to run five-mile legs and then alternate with another runner or two or three? Well, of course it would! And wouldn't you feel better knowing that you were being assisted by trusted friends and a loving family? Same answer! So, what's getting in your way?

Is it that nobody really knows, or you're not sure you trust anyone else, or no one else would be able to handle it, or that everybody has their own life? I've heard them all. How many people who know just how hard this is and who know you pretty well have asked, "What can I do?" or said, "Please call if there's anything we can do"? And how many of them have you allowed to help you and your family? For most folks, those two numbers are not the same.

If you held back because you weren't sure they really meant it when they offered to help, then do them a favor and break them of this terrible habit by actually having them do something significant. I bet 95% of them will be back for more and that's because people who care about you and your family hate feeling helpless as they watch you go through a difficult experience. As a matter of fact, there is probably nothing that gives them more pleasure than knowing that they helped you run even a short little leg of that marathon.

Knowing the Bad Spots in the Road

Unlike the marathoner who may actually get a chance to run or drive the course before the big race, you will not know where the emotional potholes will show up but you can spare yourself a great deal of worry and self-criticism by accepting that there will be lots of them.

Uncertainty, fear, fatigue, major decisions, financial challenges, and the like all have a way of destabilizing a person's emotions and can leave you feeling like you've been hit by the proverbial truck. As you travel this course a few times you will begin to learn about your own particular potholes.

For example, how do you tend to react when you have to take your child to the doctor? How do you react to a new symptom or recurrence of an old one? How do your reactions to day-to-day events change when you are sleep deprived? While eventually you may benefit from understanding where some of your more puzzling reactions come from, it can sometimes be more helpful at first to just let it happen and know that this doesn't mean that you are losing your mind. Think of it as the stretch of the course that all the marathoners hate and remember that, unless the race ends on the peak of a mountain, there have to be some downhill stretches.

The problem for you, unlike the marathoner who drove the course the day before, is that you don't know how long this stretch of the course will last until you get through it. Only when you have come out on the other side of the sadness, fear, despair, anger, and confusion, will you know that you can survive it and recognize the signs that you are heading for another difficult stretch at some later time.

The Darkest Hour

By the time you have been struggling so badly that you discovered this book on some Internet website at 2 A.M. you will likely have already traveled through some very dark emotional spots. Out of the despair of simply not knowing what to do to help your child, and/or having to face the same draining and terrifying experiences over and over again, you may have discovered that you are capable of thinking thoughts that horrify you, including negative thoughts and feelings about yourself, your spouse, the medical profession, and even your child. These are thoughts that you were sure could only be conjured up by the most tortured minds, and now they happen to be in your head.

This experience usually terrifies most people and they are sure that no one could ever understand or forgive them for such ideas. Given that conclusion, it's no surprise that they never breathe a word to anyone that they have had such thoughts and feelings. This is when the loneliness and isolation of the experience of caring for a chronically ill child or family member is the most extreme and the most damaging.

Sharing: It's Powerful Medicine

So why did you go looking for this book anyway? Chances are it was to see what someone else had to say about this reflux mess, right? And why does it matter what any of the contributors have to say? Largely because we discover that we are NOT alone. They didn't interview you for this book did they? So how could it seem like they were writing stories or thoughts straight from your own head? It's because you are not alone; your circumstances are not totally unique; your thoughts and feelings aren't crazy. There are people just like you going through difficulties with their children just like you're going through with your child.

Knowing that you are not alone is very important and powerful. And while reading stories written by others is a huge comfort, being able to converse with others through talking face to face, by phone, by letter, by email etc., is extremely important as a tool to share ideas, experiences, solutions, thoughts, and feelings. Whether that dialogue takes place with a neutral party, a trusted friend, a pastor, or the parent of a sick child is a matter of personal preference, although it often appears that the words and sentiments of those who have suffered the same challenges often seem to have the greatest credibility.

The key ingredient is the ability to say anything that's in your head, knowing that there is nothing that you have to be alone with unless you choose to do so. It is in that sharing, and the reciprocating that often comes with it, that people are able to let go of some of the extraneous emotional burden that they start carrying around as a consequence of these experiences. The marathoner can't afford to be carrying a backpack filled with unnecessary items and neither can the caregiver of a chronically ill child. Lighten your load!

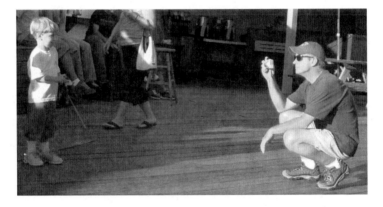

Author Dr. Richard Wirtz with Ben.

CHAPTER 10

Nutrition for the Child with Acid Reflux

Michele Innes, RD

Proper nutrition plays a key role in the care of a child with acid reflux. Such a child may be placed on a restricted diet and potentially can develop food refusals. These factors can make eating difficult and stressful for both the child and the family. Failure to thrive can result if a child's nutrition is not closely monitored during the time period he suffers from acid reflux. The goal of this chapter is to provide parents with information regarding diet and formula as well as helpful hints for introducing new foods, creating healthy eating patterns and behaviors, and participating in social events.

A gastrointestinal specialist will provide you with information regarding the diagnosis and cause of your child's reflux. There are infants who suffer from acid reflux that is non-allergy–related and then there are children who have reflux caused by food allergies. The role of a registered dietitian is to ensure that each child with acid reflux is receiving optimal nutrition to promote normal growth and development while not exacerbating the condition. Each child's nutritional care will be different based on medical need.

Non-allergy–Related Reflux

The infant or young child who suffers from non-allergy-related reflux may be placed on a formula and/or breast milk that is thickened with infant cereal. The amount of cereal per ounce of formula or breast milk is usually determined by a speech or feeding therapist and the gastrointestinal doctor. It is recommended that these babies be in an upright position during and after feedings. For infants, toddlers, and young children with reflux, it is recommended to restrict fried fatty foods, chocolate, mint, caffeine and highly acidic foods such as tomato and citrus.[1] Some of these children may benefit from being placed on reflux medications.

Allergy-Related Reflux

For the child who suffers from reflux due to food allergies, an elimination diet and a specialty formula will be part of the nutrition care plan. An elimination diet can be very successful for children with allergy-related reflux. This type of restricted diet can be very stressful for families, especially if the diet is extremely limited. Families have to be in the habit of reading labels for all purchased food items. It is critical that families call food companies to obtain product information. If information cannot be obtained then avoidance of that food is recommended. A registered dietitian will be able to provide your family with alternatives for restricted foods. Some, but not all, of these children will also require reflux medications along with an elimination diet. (The next chapter has detailed information about elimination diets.)

The nutritional status of a child with non-allergy–related or allergy-related reflux may be affected by the frequency of reflux or vomiting, poor intake due to food aversion, and the severity of diet restrictions. Infants and young children with reflux and a single food allergy can be managed well with appropriate food choices and food substitutions. However as a diet becomes more limited, the risk of dietary inadequacy increases. Your child may need to start on a specialty formula until his allergies and/or reflux improves and he is able to add more foods to his diet. A multivitamin may be added to ensure that your child is receiving all the proper vitamins and minerals.

Specialty Formulas

Table 10-1 provides specialty formula information. Your dietician or physician may recommend one of these products to deal with food allergies (Figure 10-1).

Table 10-1: Specialty Formula Information

Type of formula	Type of patient	Formula	Manufacturer
Standard	Infants who can tolerate intact cow's milk protein	Enfamil Lipil with Iron	Mead Johnson
		Similac Advance with Irion	Ross
		Good Start Supreme	Nestle
Soy-based protein	Infants who are allergic to cow's milk protein	Prosobee Lipil Isomil Advance Good Start Soy Essentials	Mead Johnson Ross Nestle
Hypo-allergenic (contain cow's milk protein that is partially broken down to make it easier to digest)	Infants who do not tolerate standard or soy-based formulas.	Pregestimil	Mead Johnson
		Nutramigen Lipil	Mead Johnson
		Alimentum Advance (also for infants with a corn allergy)	Ross
Hypo-allergenic	Children age 1–10	Peptamen Junior	Nestle
Elemental (proteins are already broken down to their simplest form, amino acids)	Infants who have severe cow's milk allergy, multiple or severe food allergies, or intolerance to soy or partially broken-down protein formulas.	Neocate Infant Formula	SHS
		Elecare	Ross
			Table continues

Table 10-1 continued			
Type of formula	**Type of patient**	**Formula**	**Manufacturer**
Elemental	Children age 1– 10	Neocate 1+ (unflavored)	SHS
		Neocate Junior (unflavored or tropical fruit flavor)	SHS
		Pediatric EO28 (juice box; orange-pineapple flavor)	SHS

* See Appendix A for manufacturers' contact information.

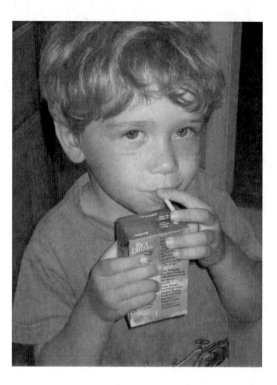

Figure 10-1. Ben substitutes rice milk for cow's milk.

When Nothing Else Works

There are children with severe dietary restrictions due to significant allergy-related reflux. Some, but certainly not all, of these children may require nutritional support by tube feedings to ensure they meet their nutritional needs. The main reasons for the initiation of a tube feeding are as follows:

- Food refusal and limited diet that result in a prolonged and inadequate intake.

- A child's need for an elemental formula, but the child is unable to take in his required amount.
- Documented failure to thrive—a child has crossed two percentiles on the growth chart. Example: a child who was originally at the 75-90 percentile for weight and within a six-month period has dropped to the 25-50 percentile.

A feeding tube is not a doctor's or registered dietitian's first option for treatment of failure to thrive. There are other options to try first such as those already discussed. However, in some cases a tube feeding is necessary to promote normal growth and development. The primary goal is to promote oral intake and then supplement as needed with tube feedings.

Re-introducing Food

Based on your doctor's and registered dietitian's recommendations, there will come a time to re-introduce food items with the hope of improving variety in your child's diet. This may be a lengthy process based on the extent to which your child's diet has been restricted. The stressful part of this process is that your child may very well react to the food being introduced, and subsequently, the reflux symptoms may reappear or worsen. It is important to understand your family limits and set reasonable goals. This may mean adding a new food for one week. If the results are positive, then you can introduce another food the following week and continue as able. In the instance where your child has reacted to the food item, return to the usual intake and wait until symptoms resolve and restart the process when you are comfortable. Be sure to carefully document all new foods tried and your child's reaction to them. This is an essential step and valuable information in figuring out what is actually happening.

It is important to give yourself permission to stop the process of trying new foods if the trials have all failed and the family is experiencing large amounts of frustration and stress. Please remember that change is a gradual process. These children experience stress, frustration and physical discomfort just like adults. You and your medical care providers need to work together as a team to make this process a positive one for your child.

Feeding Complications

The development of food aversions and feeding refusal can directly impact your child's nutritional status by decreasing his intake by mouth. There can also be a lack of progress to age-appropriate foods. Your doctor and registered dietitian may recommend an evaluation by a feeding team if they believe your child has developed these feeding complications.

Further complications can arise when a family who has an infant or young child with acid reflux does not promote normal mealtimes, patterns, and behaviors. In her book, *How to Get Your Kid to Eat...But Not Too Much*, Ellyn Satter states,

> If a child is sick, it is especially difficult, and especially important, to maintain a positive feeding relationship. Illness often requires

special feeding regimens which, in turn, put pressure on parents to take over with feeding. It doesn't work any better to be over-managing with a sick child than with a well child.[2]

Parents allowing children to get by with behavior that would normally be unacceptable is a very common issue that develops with a child suffering from reflux. Many times, parents become short-order cooks with the hope that this will increase their child's intake. In actuality, this overemphasizes the importance of eating to the child and in most cases does not improve his or her intake. It also puts more attention on food and mealtime than would normally occur.

It is essential for you as parents to enforce healthy behavior at mealtime. You should not feed a toddler on demand—instead ask him or her to come to the table with the rest of the family. Your child should have regular meals and snack times at which you prepare the foods he or she is able to eat. Your doctor and registered dietitian will be monitoring your child's growth and will provide you with alternatives if the intake is not adequate. Consistent, age-appropriate mealtime behaviors should be the constant structure around an ever-changing intake for a child with acid-reflux.

Holidays and family social events are a big part of family life. These can be very difficult for a child with reflux associated with food allergies. These events will be more enjoyable for the child if he feels like the other kids. One way of dealing with this is by addressing the food being offered prior to the social function. Family and friends will be glad to buy special foods as they are able. Parents are creative and find substitutions that are fine for their child's diet. This way the child feels included and part of the celebration.

Appendix A includes resources about food allergies and formulas. It is my hope that all the information in this chapter provides you with knowledge and guidance to assist you during this challenging time.

References

1. The Pediatric Nutrition Group of the American Dietetic Association. *Pediatric Manual of Clinical Dietetics*, 2nd edition. Chicago, IL: American Dietetic Association. 2003.

2. Satter, E. *How to Get Your Kid to Eat . . . But Not Too Much.* Palo Alto, CA: Bull Publishing Company. 1987.

CHAPTER 11

Food Allergy and Reflux

Susan Bauer, RN, MSN

"Food allergy is like religion.
Some are believers and some are not."
—Dr. Laurie Fowler

Research suggests that there may be several different causes of acid reflux. One cause, food allergy, impacts many children. Following is detailed information specific about food allergy and reflux.

Why Talk about Food Allergy in a Book about Reflux?

Reflux is a symptom. While there are many possibilities, no one is certain what causes the symptom to occur in a particular person. Reflux is a known symptom of food allergy and can make treatment a bit trickier. If you decide that allergy may be a part of the problem, make sure that you partner with a health-care provider that is a "believer" and is knowledgeable.

What Is Food Allergy?

When a child is allergic to a food, her body overreacts to one or more of the proteins in the food. The body looks at the proteins as if they are harmful invaders and produces antibodies to fight them. When your child takes in one of those foods, antibodies and histamine are released as a part of the complicated chemical reaction. If the gastrointestinal system is the "contact organ," or the part of the body that "shows" the allergic reaction, reflux or reflux-like symptoms may be the result. Researchers are finding that the allergic reaction may cause acid release and also have effects on the normal mobility of the whole gastrointestinal tract.[1] Whether this causes reflux or just adds to the symptoms has not yet been determined.

How Common are Food Allergies?

Food allergies in children vary in frequency from 6–8% in the general population. They are even a bit more common in children with frequent ear, nose, and throat illnesses and those under three years of age. Many allergists believe that the number of allergic children is on the rise.[2]

The most common food allergies in children are cow's milk, soy, eggs, wheat, corn, fish, and peanuts. Many children will outgrow these allergies by the age of five years. On the other hand, the most common adult food allergies are peanuts, tree nuts, fish, and shellfish. Adult food allergies are much less likely to resolve. Unlike other allergy-related problems such as asthma there is no specific therapy for food allergy.

What Are the Symptoms of Food Allergies?

1. Respiratory tract. Nasal obstruction, nasal drainage, sneezing, and asthma.
2. Gastrointestinal tract. Colic, gas, belching, sucking throat sounds and throat clearing, abdominal bloating or distention, acid taste, sore throat, mouth itching, heartburn, vomiting, stomach ache, diarrhea, constipation, and weight loss/failure to thrive.
3. Skin. Eczema, hives, itching, red cheeks, and other systemic symptoms.
4. Ears. Frequent ear infections and/or fluid behind the ear drum.
5. Brain and/or behavior. Headaches, learning difficulties, decreased attention, mental fatigue, sleeping difficulties, restless extremities, over activity, aggression, irritability, depression, and personality changes.
6. Miscellaneous. Joint and muscle pain, edema, fatigue, and excessive thirst.

What Are Some of the Symptoms of Reflux?

1. Hoarseness and laryngitis
2. Difficulty in eating, choking, and vomiting
3. Acid taste and heartburn

4. Excessive mucus, post nasal drip, throat clearing, and frequent swallowing
5. Chronic cough

Is All Illness Due to Food Allergy?

No, obviously there are many causes of illnesses. However, a cause of the above symptoms can be an allergy. It can be especially helpful to investigate this possibility in the child who is "always sick" or is not responding to what should be the typical treatment for a particular symptom. Those with a family history of allergies or those who look allergic are particularly in need.[3]

How Are Food Allergies Diagnosed?

Diagnosis is based on clinical symptoms and a detailed medical history, including information about allergies in the family. Allergy blood testing can sometimes be helpful, but food allergies can exist even when the blood test is negative. You may be asked to keep a food diary where you document everything your child eats for two weeks, including any symptoms you see during that period. Skin prick testing may also be used by some providers. Always remember: the human body is complicated and medical science is still developing.

How Is Food Allergy Treated?

Food avoidance is the current standard of care. Strict avoidance of a food can be extremely difficult for several reasons:

1. Poor labeling of food ingredients
2. Cross-contamination during processing
3. Milk, soy, peanuts, and eggs are found in many processed foods

Avoidance is a difficult lifestyle change for most families particularly when there are other children present in the home. Balanced nutrition can become complicated when it is necessary to remove multiple foods from the diet.

How Do I Go about a Food Avoidance Diet?

Take a deep breath. You are not alone. There are many books, newsletters, and Internet resources addressing all types of food elimination diets. Most allergists will have a handout describing how to eliminate a specific food and this will be a good place to start. Here are a few suggestions:

1. Don't try to start without making a plan.
2. If you are eliminating because of an anaphylaxis reaction, immediately remove all sources of the food from your home and make sure you have an EpiPen available.
3. Let family members, day care providers, and school personnel know, and be your child's advocate regarding his or her needs.
4. Offer to help with education and with providing snacks. Often people will want to be helpful, but won't know what is appropriate.

For other types of allergies and food eliminations, the non-emergency type:

1. Take inventory of what you usually keep on hand at home and what your typical meal plans comprise. Use your list of foods likely to contain the offending food to see what changes you will need to make.
2. Head to the grocery store and read labels.
3. Keep in mind that your child may crave the item that you are eliminating and will in some cases develop a reaction from not eating the food. This usually occurs on the third to fourth day off the food. Expect poor behavior, no matter what the age of the child.
4. On occasion you may need to cheat on the diet—there may be a birthday party or family occasion. Make sure that you get right back on the strict elimination the next day. Keep in mind that you may see symptoms or behavior changes that will go away within a few days. Sometimes you can keep the negative symptoms to a minimum by using an antihistamine just before the child indulges.
5. Most elimination diets should last for three months to start. After three months test the child's tolerance of the offending food and then wait four days between exposures. If no symptoms develop try exposing the child more frequently, i.e., three days, two days, etc. Some children will be able to go back on the food without a problem. Others may need to maintain several days between exposures. Some will have significant symptoms and need to continue the elimination.

Will the Allergy Go Away?

If the allergy produces anaphylaxis (shortness of breath, swelling in the mouth/throat, changes in blood pressure) it is considered a fixed allergy and will NOT go away. These foods must be avoided forever and your child should always have an EpiPen available in case of accidental ingestion or exposure. Other food allergies can go away over time, some within a few months and some may take several years.

Terms to Know

Allergy. Reaction of the body caused by the immune system, which sees common substances, either environmental or eaten, as something "bad" and trying to "invade" the body. Reactions are developed through repetitive exposure. In children, dust and foods tend to be the most common allergies.

Anaphylaxis. An immediate response to food protein that typically produces respiratory distress, throat/tongue swelling, and blood pressure problems, and requires emergency treatment.

Hypersensitivity. An abnormal reaction from eating, drinking, or ingesting a food. The reaction could be due to food allergy or intolerance.

Intolerance. Some consider all reactions that are not anaphylaxis to be food intolerance rather than a true allergy. This may include food reactions that occur within 15 minutes and up to two days after ingestion.

Can We Prevent Food Allergies?

When one parent has a food allergy the risk that his or her child will develop allergies is almost double. We would say that the child has allergic tendencies and he or she may or may not have the same food allergies as the parent(s). Some of the following suggestions may help reduce food allergies.

1. Prevent allergies prenatally. Some research suggests that limiting a pregnant woman's intake of allergenic foods can help prevent allergy in the infant. Avoiding foods such as milk/dairy, peanuts, or shellfish could be helpful.
2. Breastfeed as long as possible. Breast milk is rich in the immunoglobulin IgA which acts as a protective coating in the intestines preventing food allergens from entering the blood stream.
3. Delay introduction of solid foods. Mature intestines are better able to keep food proteins from entering the blood stream which may lead to the development of antibodies to the food proteins. It is recommended that you wait until 18 months of age before introducing potentially allergenic foods such as egg whites, tomatoes, shellfish, and peanut butter.
4. Rotate the diet. Keeping lots of variety in the diet will limit the exposure of any particular food and therefore limit the development of a food-antibody response. Food allergies are dose related.

Frequently Asked Questions
Is milk allergy the same as lactose intolerance? No, they are not the same. Lactose intolerance occurs when an enzyme that breaks down lactose is missing from the

bowel. It can be treated by taking an oral form of the enzyme or using dairy products that have lactase added. Milk allergy is an allergy to one or more of the cow's milk proteins. Those proteins are present in all milk, no matter what the fat content.

Is goat milk okay? Goat milk protein is very similar to cow milk protein and therefore is not recommended.

My child drinks a lot of milk and eats a lot of cheese. How can he be allergic? Children will often crave the foods they are allergic to because endorphins are released as part of the allergic reaction. The endorphins make them feel good, but then the other allergy symptoms make them feel bad. They keep going back to the same food to get that good feeling and the cycle continues. This cycle can wear down the body and prevent a person from feeling the full allergic reaction to a particular food. Removing a food from the diet for at least four days will often bring out the body's true reaction to that food. This is called a food withdrawal/challenge.

What can I substitute for milk/dairy? Infants and toddlers should drink a hypo-allergenic formula. Please talk with your health-care provider about this. They need the nutrients that are present in the formulas but may not like the taste. Older children can use rice milk. It is best not to use soy milk on a daily basis, because it could lead to a soy allergy and soy is extremely difficult to avoid.

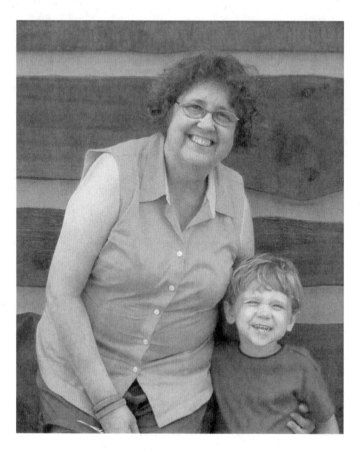

Author Susan Bauer with Ben.

References
1. Hill, D.J. Gastroesophageal reflux and food allergy. *Focus on Food Allergy in Childhood.*
http://72.14.203.104/search?q=cache:Tto6o543uswJ
:www.shsweb.co.uk/neocate/prof/docs/boston%2520pro.pdf+%2

2Hill,+D.J.%22++%22focus+on+food+allergy%22&hl=en&gl=us&
ct=clnk&cd=1&client=safari. (Accessed 2001).

2. National Institute of Health. Report of the expert panel on
food allergy research. http://www.niaid.nih.gov/dait/pdf/11-20-
03FAreport1.pdf. (Accessed 2003.)

3. Rapp, D. *Is This Your Child: Discovering and Treating
Unrecognized Allergies in Children and Adults.* Quill, NY: William
Morrow & Co. 2003.

4. Nowak-Wegrzyn, A. Future approaches to food allergy.
Pediatrics. 111, 6 (June 2003): 1672-80.

5. Sampson, H. Update on Food Allergy, *The Journal of Allergy and Clinical Immunology* 113, 5 (2004) 805-819.

CHAPTER 12

Extra-Esophageal Reflux and Symptoms of the Ear, Nose, and Throat

Marcella Bothwell, MD; Jeff Phillips, PharmD; and Stacy Turpin, MS

Intermittent reflux of stomach contents into the esophagus is a normal physiological process that occurs because of transient relaxation of the sphincter located where the esophagus connects to the stomach. Gastroesophageal reflux is considered to be abnormal or pathologic if it produces symptoms, and is then referred to as gastroesophageal reflux disease (GERD).

GERD is a well-documented and common occurrence among adults, but during the last twenty years, it has been increasingly recognized as a clinical entity among children and infants. GERD most commonly results in vomiting, abdominal or chest pain, heartburn, arousal from sleep, and regurgitation (spitting up).

If gastric reflux reaches the level of the pharynx (throat) by moving past both the lower and upper esophageal sphincters (Figure 12-1), it is termed extra-esophageal reflux (EER). Evidence is accumulating that EER can be a factor in disorders of the upper and lower airway in both adults and children.[1,2]

Infants may be especially predisposed to reflux-related problems because they have relatively more reflux events than adults. In a survey of 948 infants, it was found that nearly 50% of babies less than 3 months old had reflux events that resulted in regurgitation or spitting up at least once a day.[3] The number increased to a maximum of 67% of 4-month-olds. By 1 year of age, the percent of infants with daily regurgitation events was less than 5%.

Although symptoms of GERD are fairly easy to diagnose, extra-esophageal reflux is a more difficult diagnosis. "Silent reflux," or atypical reflux in which the patient has no gastrointestinal symptoms, is very common in children with upper and lower airway complaints. Determining the involvement of EER requires verifying its presence by some diagnostic methodology.

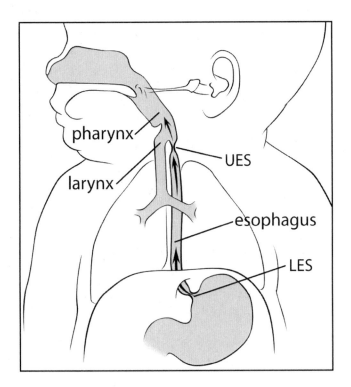

Figure 12-1. How extra-esophageal reflux arises. Arrows show path of reflux out of the stomach. UES = upper esophageal sphincter and LES = lower esophageal sphincter.

A methodology commonly used to determine whether a person has gastroesophageal reflux is to measure acidity by means of a pH-detecting "probe" placed at the lower esophageal sphincter (LES). However, traditional pH probes placed to detect acid reflux at the LES can easily overlook EER in the child. A significant percentage of children who have EER show normal pH data from probes placed at the LES.[4,5] Therefore, a better approach to EER diagnosis is to monitor pH in the pharynx or upper esophagus. Although pharyngeal probes provide excellent measures of EER, they are uncomfortable for some children because the procedure involves insertion of rubber tubing through the nose. Parents also shy away, especially once they learn the tubing must stay in the nose for 24 hours.

An innovative alternative for diagnosing EER is the Bravo pH capsule. This capsule is wireless, and is placed in the upper esophagus just behind the upper esophageal sphincter.[6] The probe then transmits data to a wireless receiver. It is then complied and analyzed. The Bravo system has been a very good way to measure upper esophageal reflux without any tubing.

In this chapter we focus on how EER results in damage to cells and tissues of the larynx and upper respiratory tract. We also discuss a number of ear, nose, throat, and laryngeal disorders commonly encountered in pediatric patients and examine evidence for the role of EER in causing or exacerbating these conditions.

How Reflux Affects the Airway

The larynx, or voice box, acts as a two-way valve to prevent aspiration of food and liquids into the lungs during swallowing. During breathing, the larynx is open, allowing air to move in and out of the lungs via the trachea, but during swallowing, the larynx functions to close off the airway.

Even so, the proximity of the airway to the esophageal entrance makes the potential for reflux to enter the airway very high in certain situations. When a person is lying flat, refluxing gastric contents can readily flow into the esophagus to the level of the larynx and throat. Babies are especially prone to EER because their lower esophageal sphincter does not reach maturity until 18 months and therefore does not always function fully to keep gastric contents in the stomach.

Acid and the digestive enzyme pepsin are responsible for the damaging effects of reflux. Stomach tissue is most protected against their damaging effects, but even so, erosions and ulcers can develop. While not nearly as resistant to the effects of acid and pepsin as the stomach tissue, the esophagus is adapted to handle some acid exposure that occurs due to intermittent physiological reflux. Peristalsis, which is the rhythmic, wavelike movement of the esophagus, helps push reflux back into the stomach (Figure 12-2A). The esophagus secretes mucus that forms a protective barrier against the corrosive effects of the reflux. The esophagus is also lined by a specialized layer of cells called stratified squamous epithelium that secretes bicarbonate ions, which can neutralize the acid (Figure 12-2B and 12-2C). Even with these protective mechanisms in place, acid may still penetrate the epithelial layers and irritate nerve endings, which results in the sensation of "heartburn."

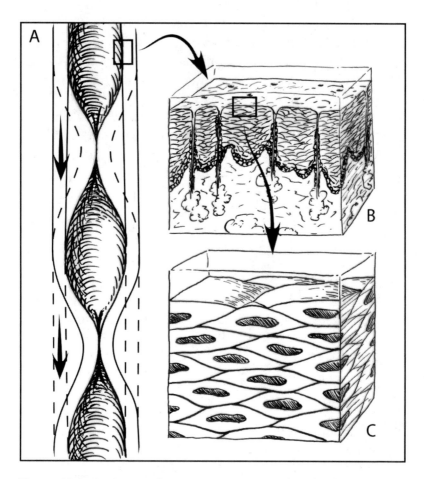

Figure 12-2. Acid-protective mechanisms of the esophagus. A. Peristalsis pushes gastric contents back into the stomach. B. Esophageal epithelium contains glands that secrete a protective layer of mucus. C. Layers of stratified squamous epithelial cells secrete acid-neutralizing bicarbonate ions.

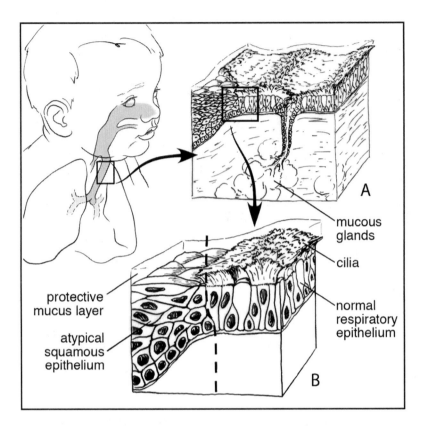

Figure 12-3. Cellular structure of the upper respiratory tract.
A. Respiratory epithelium. B. Transformation of ciliated epithelial
cells to unciliated squamous cells in response to EER.

Unlike the stomach and esophagus, the respiratory tract
is extremely sensitive to the damaging effects of gastric
fluids. The respiratory tract is lined by a cell layer called
pseudo-stratified, ciliated columnar epithelium, which is
very different in structure from the epithelium in the
esophagus (Figure 12-3). Respiratory epithelia possess
tiny hairs called cilia that perform a protective function.
The sweeping action of the cilia keeps the airway clear

by removing mucus from the respiratory tract. The cilia also help eliminate infectious and allergenic materials from the body because any bacteria, viruses, dust, pollen or mold that float onto the cilia also are swept out of the airway.

When repeatedly exposed to reflux, the respiratory columnar epithelium sometimes will change into stratified squamous epithelium like that found in the esophagus. Although more resistant to the damaging effects of reflux, squamous cells do not possess cilia. By causing the loss of cilia, EER compromises an essential cleansing process in the respiratory tract.

Sometimes when explaining to patients the difference between the ability of the esophagus and the airway to tolerate reflux, we use the analogy of the esophagus being a rubber hose and the airway being tissue paper. While not entirely accurate, it does paint a picture of the relative sensitivities of the two.

Although direct irritation of the respiratory tract by acid and pepsin can bring about the signs and symptoms of airway disease, reflux can also have an indirect, or referred, effect on the airway even if it never leaves the esophagus. This indirect effect occurs because the esophagus and airway are connected to a common central nerve called the vagus. When acid refluxing into the lower esophagus interacts with special structures called receptors, nerve impulses can arc backwards along the vagus to cause spastic closure of the larynx (laryngospasm).This reflexive response of the airway to reflux is yet another way in which the body protects itself from aspiration.

Common Ear, Nose, and Throat Conditions Resulting from EER

A number of ear, nose, and throat disorders commonly encountered in children and infants have been found to be associated with EER. For some disorders, the association is likely causative, that is, the acid and pepsin in reflux are directly responsible for the signs and symptoms associated with the condition. For other disorders, EER is not necessarily causative, but the presence of reflux can make the signs and symptoms much worse. In a few cases, it has been speculated that symptoms worsen because the condition increases the likelihood that reflux can escape the esophagus and get into the airway. In other words, rather than EER causing the condition, the condition causes EER. This section provides an overview of the signs and symptoms of laryngeal and upper airway disorders commonly encountered in pediatric practice, and how EER can bring about or aggravate these disorders. The role of anti-reflux therapy in treating these conditions is also discussed.

Effects of EER on the larynx. The larynx is anatomically just in front of the esophagus and therefore is very susceptible to the effects of EER. Multiple sites of the larynx can be irritated and cause a number of different signs and symptoms. Some of these include chronic cough, hoarseness with or without vocal cord nodules, laryngeal ulcers, and vocal cord dysfunction.

Cough is one sign commonly associated with irritation of the larynx. Cough is a protective reflex that removes irritants or infectious organisms such as those causing pneumonia. Irritants are detected by *cough receptors*, which are nerve endings located in the larynx and other parts of the respiratory tree. Receptors are also located in the naso- and oropharynx, the sinuses, and the ears.[7] Through coughing, the airway tries to relieve itself of its acid load as best as it can. However, persistent cough can itself further irritate the airway. EER is an important agent in *chronic cough*, which is coughing that continues for 3–8 weeks. Excluding infectious diseases, EER is third most common cause of chronic cough in children and the most common cause in infants up to 18 months old.[8]

Hoarseness is another sign that can be associated with the deleterious effects of reflux on the larynx. Hoarseness is a general term for any abnormal voice quality, but voice quality can be further described as breathy or harsh, husky or rough, strident, or coarse. Though voice intensity varies with the amount of air pressure against vocal cord resistance, voice quality is primarily determined by length, tension, strength of movement, mass, or position of the vocal chords.[9] Any aberration of length or tension of the vibrating segment, mass, posture, or strength of the vocal cords may result in hoarseness. In a study of children aged 2–12 years old who had chronic hoarseness for more than 6 months, 70% of them were found to also have GERD.[9] When researchers directly examined the vocal cords of these children, one child's vocal cords looked normal, but the remainder had a variety of abnormalities that included cord swelling, nodules (Figure 12-4), and evidence of healing ulcerations.

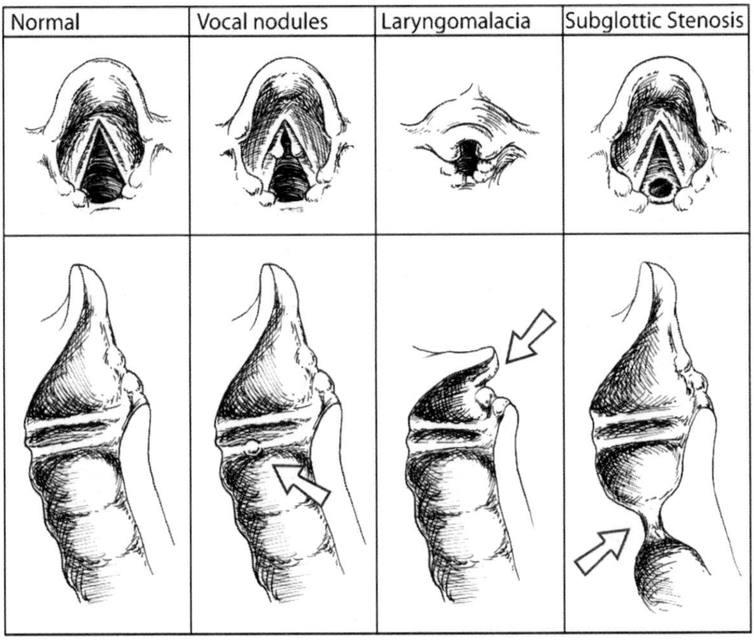

Figure 12-4. Top and side views of the larynx afflicted with EER-associated conditions compared to a normal larynx. Top views are what an ENT physician would see looking down a child's throat using a laryngoscope. Arrows point to affected regions: vocal nodules are swellings on the vocal cords; in laryngomalacia, the tissues at the entrance to the larynx collapse upon inhaling; subglottic stenosis is a narrowing of the area below the vocal cords.

Another abnormality of the vocal cords that can be associated with damage from reflux is paradoxical vocal cord dysfunction (PVCD). During breathing, normally functioning vocal cords should move into an open position to allow free flow of air through the larynx. In PVCD, the vocal cords are inappropriately closed with breathing. When cord movement is not synchronous with breathing, voice quality is not affected, but it creates a sensation of airway obstruction. PVCD can be quite distressing and mimic asthma or severe inspiratory airway obstruction. In rare cases, it has resulted in placement of a tracheotomy tube to assist breathing. PVCD is most commonly found in teenagers,[10] but cases masquerading as bilateral vocal cord paralysis have been reported in newborns.[11] Reflux therapy resolves PVCD and may be curative.[10,12]

Another sign of a problem in the airway is stridor, which is a coarse, high-pitched sound heard when inhaling. This noise results from turbulent, rapid air flow through a narrowed portion of the airway. Because a number of airway disorders can cause stridor, a physician should explore all possibilities when evaluating patients, but EER may play a significant role in those conditions most commonly associated with stridor.

Airway abnormalities present at birth are responsible for 87% of stridor cases in infants.[11] The most common of these congenital abnormalities is laryngomalacia.[11] Laryngomalacia refers to an abnormal floppiness of the laryngeal tissues just forward of the vocal cords at the airway entrance. Stridor results because upon inspiration, these floppy tissues get pulled into opening of the airway, narrowing the diameter of the opening by partially blocking it (see Figure 12-4). Although inspiratory breathing is noisy, breathing on expiration is normal, as is the voice.

Parents may notice their baby has noisy breathing at birth, but usually laryngomalacia-associated stridor becomes most noticeable at 1–2 months when the infant is becoming more active and making more demands on the airway. Respiratory effort and noisy breathing typically get worse before they resolve, usually by 18 months of age.

Two studies have shown a strong association between laryngomalacia and gastroesophageal reflux. In one study, 80% of infants with stridor due to laryngomalacia also had gastroesophageal reflux.[12] In another, more recent study, the severity of laryngomalacia was shown to be directly related to the severity of gastroesophageal reflux.[13]

The co-association of laryngomalacia and reflux may be a common manifestation of neuromuscular immaturity that simultaneously results in flaccid airway structures and poor esophageal sphincter tone,[12] which may explain why symptoms often disappear as the child matures. Another possibility is that EER is a secondary effect of the laryngomalacia in which the inspiration of air against the narrowed airway creates a suction effect that pulls reflux up and out of the esophagus.[12] Either way, reflux can cause a worsening of symptoms of laryngomalacia because the inflammation and swelling of the laryngeal tissues result in still greater obstruction of the airway. Aggressive reflux therapy is recommended.[5]

Reflux may also play a role in children who suffer from repeated cases of croup. Symptoms of croup include stridor, a barking cough, hoarseness, and difficulty breathing. In children older than a year, an isolated case of croup often comes on the heels of an upper respiratory infection and is usually caused by a virus-induced inflammation of the larynx. However, infants less than 1 year old who have repeated cases of croup may have condition called subglottic stenosis (SGS), which is an abnormal narrowing of the subglottis, a region of the larynx located below the vocal cords (see Figure 12-4). Different severities of SGS exist and are graded 1–4, with a grade 1 being the least severe and grade 4 representing nearly complete obstruction of the airway.

Infants can be born with SGS, but they can also develop it from physical injury to the larynx. Physical injury includes damage caused by acid reflux. Studies in animals in which direct application of acid to the larynx resulted in the formation of SGS confirms a causal association between EER and acquired SGS.[14] One study has shown that infants who have recurrent cases of severe croup requiring hospitalization are more likely to have an additional diagnosis of reflux,[15] and another reported that 80% of children undergoing surgery to repair their SGS had at least one positive test for EER.[16]

A mild, grade-1 SGS that would normally not be noticed can be exacerbated by EER or recurrent viral illness. Children with grade-1 SGS may spontaneously improve as they get older, and often anti-reflux medication is all that is needed to keep the airway sufficiently open until the SGS resolves. Severe SGS requires surgical intervention, but anti-reflux medications help improve the success rate of these surgeries and reduce the need for additional operations, presumably because healing can occur more readily in the absence of acid.[17]

Effects of EER on the pharynx, sinuses, and ears.
Not only can EER irritate the larynx, it can also irritate the pharynx. Reflux can flow up into the oro- and naso-pharynx and may even reach the nasal and sinus cavities (Figure 12-5). EER has accordingly been implicated in a number of symptoms and disorders of the pharynx, nose, sinuses, and ears. Pharyngeal signs and symptoms associated with or caused by EER include: sensations of choking or a lump in the throat with or without constant throat clearing, adenoid enlargement, rhinosinusitis, eustachian tube dysfunction, and middle ear infections.

Inflammation of the pharynx can result in globus pharyngeus, which is the medical term for having a sensation of a lump in the throat.[18] The sensation is most notable between swallows. EER is the most common underlying factor, although other anatomical, physiological, and psychological factors should be considered.

Enlarged adenoids, which can block the nasal airway, may also be attributable to EER in very young children. In a study of children less than 2 years old who underwent surgery for removal of enlarged adenoids, 42% also had a GERD diagnosis. By contrast, GERD was diagnosed in only 7% of a control group of children getting surgery for insertion of ear tubes but whose adenoids were normal. The association between reflux and

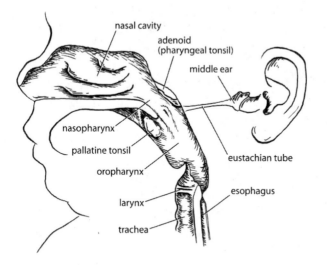

Figure12-5. Due to the close proximity of the esophagus to the airway, EER can get into the larynx, the pharynx, and even into eustachian tubes that connect to the ears.

adenoid enlargement was even stronger in children age 1 or less. In this age group, 88% of those requiring an adenoidectomy had a GERD diagnosis, whereas only 14% of the control group getting ear tubes had a GERD diagnosis.[19]

Reflux may be a factor in inflammation of the nose and sinuses. Called rhinosinusitis, this inflammation is caused by obstruction of the final common pathway of the maxillary, ethmoid, and frontal sinus tracts (Figure 12-6). Although infection is often present, it is not typically the primary underlying factor for rhinosinusitis. Rather, infection occurs secondarily because the impaired drainage due to swelling, or edema, of sinus and

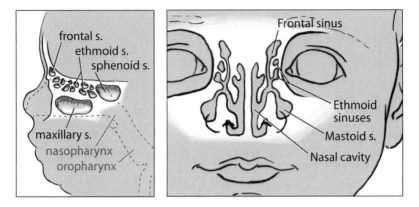

Figure 12-6. Front and side views of the sinus cavities. These cavities, which are located in the bones of the face are connected to the nasal cavity by narrow passages. EER can cause inflammation of the sinuses. Infection is often a secondary complication.

nasal tissues creates an ideal environment for the growth of bacteria. Anything irritating the sinus and nasal tissues can result in swelling of tissues: allergies, cigarette smoke, recurrent viral infections, and EER. Edema from EER is a common cause of sinus obstruction.[20] People with chronic sinus problems often have corrective surgery. However, one study found that 89% of children who underwent reflux therapy in addition to maximal medical management of allergy and other irritants could avoid sinus surgery.[21]

Like the sinuses, the ear has natural openings that must remain functional to prevent problems. As in rhinosinusitis, the development of middle ear infections (otitis media) is a secondary complication that results from impaired function of the eustachian tube. Studies using animals as models have shown that exposure of the middle ear and the eustachian tube to acid and pepsin results in failure of the eustachian tube to perform its dual function of sweeping out secretions and modulating pressure within the ear.[22,23] In a study examining patients who had chronic ear problems, treatment with the anti-reflux medication omeprazole resulted in complete resolution of symptoms.[24]

Conclusion

EER is a topic to be investigated along with other important causes of ENT problems such as allergy, immune deficiency, smoke exposure, and other yet-to-be defined factors. EER sometimes is a difficult diagnosis to make and is even more difficult if not suspected. However, if EER is discovered to be an underlying or contributing problem, instituting reflux therapy often can control or even eliminate symptoms altogether.

Acknowledgment. The authors thank Pamela S. Cooper, PhD, for writing and editorial assistance in revising the manuscript.

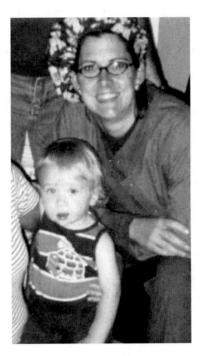

Co-author Dr. Marcy Bothwell with Ben.

References

1. Rosbe, K.W., M. Kenna, and A.D. Auerback. Extraesophageal reflux in pediatric patients with upper respiratory symptoms. *Arch Otolaryngol Head Neck Surg* 129 (Nov 2003): 1213-20.

2. DeVault, K.R. Extraesophageal symptoms of GERD. *Cleve Clin J Med* 70, suppl 5 (2003):S20-S32.

3. Nelson, S., E. Chen, G. Syniar, and K. Christoffel. Prevalence of symptoms of gastroesophageal reflux during infancy: a pediatric practice-based survey. *Arch Pediatr Adolesc Med* 151 (June 1997): 569-72.

4. Little, J.P., B.L.Matthews, M.S. Glock Koufman JA, Reboussin DM, Loughlin CJ, McGuirt WF Jr. Extraesophageal pediatric reflux: 24-hour double-probe pH monitoring of 222 children. *Ann Otol Rhinol Laryngol* 169, suppl (1997): 1-16.

5. Mathews, B.L., J.P., Little, McGuirt, W.F., Jr., and J.A. Koufman. Reflux in infants with laryngomalacia: results of 24-hour double-probe pH monitoring. *Otolaryngol Head Neck Surg* 120 (June, 1999): 860-4.

6. Bothwell, M.R., J. Phillips, and S. Bauer. Upper esophageal pH monitoring of children with the Bravo pH capsule. *Laryngoscope* 114 (April 2004): 768-8.

7. Irwin, R.S., L.P. Boulet, M.M. Cloutier, Fuller R, Gold PM, Hoffstein V, Ing AJ, McCool FD, O'Byrne P, Poe RH, Prakash UB, Pratter MR, Rubin BK.. Managing cough as a defense mechanism and as a symptom: a consensus panel report of the American College of Chest Physicians. *Chest* 114, 2 suppl managing (1998): 133S-181S.

8. Holinger. L.D., and A.D. Sanders. Chronic cough in infants and children: an update. *Laryngoscope* 101 (June 1991): 596-605.

9. Kalach. N., L. Gumpert, P. Contencin, and C. Dupont. Dual-probe pH monitoring for the assessment of gastroesophageal reflux in the course of chronic hoarseness in children. *Turk J Pediatr* 42 (Jul-Sep 2000): 186-91.

10. Powell, D.M., Bll. Karanfilov, K.B. Beechler, K. Treole, M.D. Trudeau, and L.A. Forrest. Paradoxical vocal cord dysfunction in juveniles. *Arch Otolaryngol Head Neck Surg* 126 (2000):22:29-34.

11. Heatley, D.G., and E. Swift. Paradoxical vocal cord dysfunction in an infant with stridor and gastresophageal reflux. *Int J Pediatr Otorhinolaryngol* 34 (Jan 1996): 149-51.

12. Belmont, J.R., and K. Grundfast. Congenital laryngeal stridor (laryngomalacia): etiologic factors and associated disorders. *Ann Otol Rhinol Laryngol* 93 (1984):51: 430-7.

13. Giannoni, C., M. Sulek, E.M. Friedman, and N.O. Duncan, III. Gastroesophageal reflux association with laryngomalacia: a prospective study. *Int J Pediatr Otorhinolaryngo* 43 (Feb1998): 11-20.

14. Little, F.B., J.A. Koufman, R.I Kohut, and R.B. Marshall. Effect of gastric acid on the pathogenesis of subglottic stenosis. *Ann Otol Rhinol Laryngol* 94 (1985): 51:516-9.

15. Waki E.Y., D.N. Madgy, W.M. Belenky, and V.C. Gower. The incidence of gastroesophageal reflux in recurrent croup. *Int J Pediatr Otorhino-laryngol* 32 (Jul 1995): 223-32.

16. Yellon, R. M. Parameswaran, and B. Brandom. Decreasing morbidity following laryngotracheal reconstruction in children. *Int J Ped Otorhinolaryngol* (Aug 1997): 145-54.

17. Halstead, L.A. Role of gastroesophageal reflux in pediatric upper airway disorders. *Otolaryngol Head Neck Surg* 120 (Feb 1999): 208-14.

18. Bluestone, CD, Stool S, Kenna, M, et al., ed. *Pediatric Otolaryngology*. 4th ed. Philadelphia:Saunders; 2003.

19. Carr, M.M., C.P., Poje, D. Ehrig, and L.S. Brodsky. Incidence of reflux in young children undergoing adenoidectomy. *Laryngoscope* 111 (Dec 2001): 2170-2.

20. Loehrl, T.A., and T.L. Smith. Chronic sinusitis and gastroesophageal reflux: are the related? *Curr Opin Otolaryngol Head Neck Surg* 12 (Feb 2004): 18-20.

21. Bothwell, M.R., D.S. Parsons, A. Talbot, G.J. Barbero, and B. Wilder. Outcome of reflux therapy on pediatric chronic sinusitis. *Otolaryngol Head Neck Surg* 121(Sep 1999): 255-62.

22. White, D.R., S.B. Heavner, S.M. Hardy, and J. Prazma. Gastroesophageal reflux and Eustachian tube dysfunction in an animal model. *Laryngoscope* 112 (Jun 2002): 955-61.

23. Heavner, S.B., S.M. Hardy, D.R. White, C.T. McQueen, j. Prazma, and H.C. Pillsbury, III. Function of the Eustachian tube after weekly exposure to pepsin/hydrochloric acid. *Otolaryngol Head Neck Surg* 125 (Sep 2001): 123-9.

24. Poelmans, J., J. Tack, and L. Feenstra. Prospective study on the incidence of chronic ear complaints related to gastroesophageal reflux and on the outcome of antireflux therapy. *Ann Otol Rhinol Laryngol* 111 (Oct 2002): 933-8.

CHAPTER 13

The Use of Medications in Acid Reflux Disease

Jeff Phillips, PharmD, and Stacy Turpin, MS

The reflux of gastric contents is a well-documented and common occurrence among adults. During the last twenty years, gastroesophageal reflux disease (GERD) has been increasingly recognized as a clinical problem among children. Several investigators have noted that approximately one-half of all newborns have reflux.[1,2] In one study the peak incidence of reflux occurred at approximately 4 months of age. Approximately 70% of these infants exhibited signs of reflux disease.[2]

Left untreated, gastroesophageal reflux most commonly results in vomiting (spitting up), abdominal or chest pain, heartburn, arousal from sleep, and regurgitation. [3,4] Studies have found that up to 75% of patients with symptoms of upper and/or lower respiratory tract disorders such as asthma, croup, bronchitis, pneumonia, sinusitis, laryngomalacia, and subglottic stenosis have reflux disease.[5-22] Gastroesophageal reflux may also be associated with more serious complications such as apparent life-threatening events, isolated bradycardia with irregular respiratory efforts, apnea, hypotension, reduced cerebral blood flow, and sudden infant death syndrome (SIDS). [3,23-28] In a study of 14 infants hospitalized for respiratory distress and recurrent apnea, one study found all the patients to have positive reflux testing results.

The treatment of acid reflux disease in children is a good example of how easily things can go wrong when:

1. the condition, or its symptoms, are not readily obvious (atypical in the way it presents),
2. a diagnosis requires a test (pH study) administered by a specialist (pediatric gastroenterologist), and
3. there exists a number of safe medicines available to treat the disease/condition but these medicines have been poorly studied in the population of interest (infants and children).

The above combination can seem to wreak havoc on the ability of physicians to figure out what to do and when to do it. Here is a real-life example:

A mother who already has a 4-year-old daughter brings her 6-month-old son in to see the pediatrician with a chief complaint of nighttime wakening and the inability to console the baby. In other words, the baby cries a lot and the mother cannot seem to get him to stop. The pediatrician is likely to have little to go on at this point and discusses behavioral issues with the mom. "Little babies may cry at night but you should let them cry and they will go back to sleep. It is okay to check on them to make sure they haven't gotten caught in the bedding, but just let them cry."

The mother is thinking to herself, "I know this; I've raised a child already." However, the mother is reluctant to challenge the pediatrician and agrees to try this even though she has already been doing this. She waits through a week of frustration and calls the pediatrician back. She speaks to the nurse who tells her to try for another week or so. The mother has not been sleeping and the father has not been helping much but knows that there is a problem. The mother is frustrated—beyond frustrated—as weeks turn into months. Her child is taking only an ounce or two at a feeding—very slowly.

When the mother finally gets back in to see the pediatrician, she is sent to a behavioral or feeding specialist. This goes on awhile and the child develops an ear infection, which leads to treatment with antibiotics. This causes bad diaper rash and Candida (a yeast infection in the child's throat) which further worsens the feeding problem. The child has very hard and irregular stools which further worries the mother. The child seems to get a lot of respiratory tract infections or at least is coughing a lot with a chronic runny nose. The mother finally gets back to see the pediatrician who considers that the child may have some type of immune deficiency. This leads to more tests and all the while the child does not seem one bit better.

The stress of the situation and the mother's sleep deprivation causes strain on the parents' relationship. The mother is near her limit and does not know where to turn to next. And in the middle of this already stressful situation, the child has an event where he turns blue and stops breathing. The mother panics and takes the child to the emergency room. The child spontaneously recovers breathing prior to arrival at the hospital. The physician at the emergency room states that the child might have asthma or may have had a seizure or an apneic event. This happens again one week later and the physician decides to keep the child in the hospital for a complete work up. These are difficult days with EEGs, EKGs, blood draws, tests, and more tests.

Because she was not getting the answers to her son's symptoms, the mother did some Internet research and thinks her child may have reflux. She mentions this to her pediatrician while at the hospital. The pediatrician reluctantly agrees to consult a gastroenterologist (peds GI). The pediatric specialist evaluates the child. He wants to do a test called a pH probe study.

A week later the parents bring the now eight-month-old child into the hospital for the pH study. The peds GI puts the child in a room without the parents. The baby is screaming and the mother is crying. The child comes out in about one hour, sedated, with a tube coming out of his nose and his hands taped on restraints so that he does not pull the tube out of his nose—which is exactly what any of us would try to do if we were eight months old. The child wakes up and becomes more active and begins to cry. The peds GI tells the mother that the tube is running into the nose and then into the esophagus and will have to stay in for 24 hours in order to get good information about the acid.

About an hour later the parents are thinking there is no way they can do this for 24 hours. Their son is fighting the restraints and is trying to pull out the tube (even though it is taped to his nose). The parents loosen the restraints a bit and things seem a little better. A few hours later the child pulls the tube out. The mother doesn't know what to do. She calls the peds GI who tells her to come into the office. She goes to the office and he tells her he will download the information and there may be enough data to make a diagnosis.

However, the results of the pH probe study are determined to be inconclusive. The peds GI puts the child on Zantac®. The next day things seem better as the boy sleeps six hours during the night. This is the first time this has happened since he was 2 1/2 months old. The parents are really excited but exhausted. Then a week passes and things remain good. However, on the tenth day of Zantac®, things go bad. The child seems to be regressing. The mother calls the peds GI who increases the dose of Zantac®. This seems to help for a few days but then the regression occurs again. The reflux symptoms (mostly crying, and not taking the bottle again) increase each day.

The peds GI adds Prevacid® SoluTab 15mg (1/2 tablet) to take in the morning. This is hard for the parents to give because it contains little pellets that the child seems to have trouble swallowing. However, the parents try to make sure that the boy gets the 1/2 tablet each morning. The mother puts it in a little water and even though the little pellets seem to always end up on his lips she scoops them back into his mouth. It is difficult but she does it because she doesn't know what else to do. The next week things really get worse and the parents think they are right back where they were before the Zantac® started working. They contact the peds GI who has an opening in two weeks. In the meantime he tells them to give the Prevacid® SoluTab and add Pepcid® twice per day. This does not seem to have any effect. He adds sucralfate four times per day. This also has no effect.

Finally the parents go in to see the peds GI and he thinks that it may not be reflux but it might be eosinophilic esosphagitis. He suggests that he would like to take a look in the esophagus and get some biopsies. The parents don't know what this is but they don't really know what else to do. A lot of time has passed, with a lot of difficult times and no definitive answers.

Although this may sound like it is a very unlikely scenario I speak to mothers at least once a week who have gone through this and worse. One major problem with the preceding scenario is that the child had atypical symptoms of acid reflux. You see, the *typical* symptom of acid reflux is a burning pain in the esophagus. All the other symptoms are atypical. Some atypical symptoms* include:

1. Apnea followed by bradycardia (slowing of heart rate)
2. Asthma
3. SIDS (sudden infant death syndrome)
4. Acute Life Threatening Events (ALTEs): i.e., "stops breathing and turns blue"
5. Recurrent otitis media (ear infections)
6. Coughing
7. Hoarseness
8. Recurrent pneumonia
9. Chronic infection
10. Sinusitis
11. Persistent crying (inconsolable): i.e., "colic-like behavior"
12. Nighttime awakening (crying and crying, inconsolable)
13. Failure to thrive
14. Seizures
15. Feeding abnormalities (e.g., only takes an ounce at a feeding)
16. Back arching behavior (appears to be a seizure)

---

* Note, if your child is not able to communicate (e.g., under 1 year of age) then he or she is not able to let anyone know of the pain, thus crying is a natural response (i.e., his or her way of communicating).

The Use of Medicines in Acid Reflux Disease

Children are usually the last group to be studied with regard to medicines, not just medicines for acid reflux but medicines in general. This means that doctors end up with a lack of:

1. information about how to properly use medicine in children, and
2. formulations that are specifically made for children (e.g., liquids or chewable products that make compliance possible and in dosage strengths for children).

This problem is recognized by the Food and Drug Administration (FDA). The FDA makes it easy and attractive for drug companies to study their medicines in children after the medicines have already been approved in adults. First, if the pharmacokinetics (i.e., the way the medicine is absorbed and moves around in the body, and how the body removes the medicine) can be shown to be similar in adults and children, then typically no further studies are requested by the FDA.

Second, once the pediatric studies are accepted by the FDA and the medicine is approved for use in children, the FDA gives the drug company an extra 6 months of patent protection for the medicine (in all of its uses, not just in children).

It would seem that there would be quite a lot of pediatric approvals of medicines occurring, but this is not the case. Often, the drug companies that do take advantage of this opportunity wait until the medicine is about to run out of patent protection or until one of its competitors gets approval first. For an example related to acid reflux medications and proton pump inhibitors (PPI), Astra Zeneca—makers of Prilosec® (omeprazole)—did not get a pediatric approval for Prilosec® until the last year of its patent. The only other company to get pediatric approval for a PPI is TAP—makers of Prevacid® (lansoprazole), which gained pediatric approval following Astra Zeneca's lead.

What is more distressing is that the FDA-approved label for using Prilosec® in children did not become available until after Astra Zeneca's new drug, Nexium®, had already been released on the market. Further, Nexium® has been available for several years and yet there are no data or approvals for pediatric use.

As mentioned above, none of these medicines is available in a dosage form that is acceptable for young children (i.e., a liquid without enteric-coated granules). More recently, a true liquid form of omeprazole has become available as an FDA-approved medicine. It is trade named Zegerid®. Since omeprazole is approved for use in children it is reasonable to use Zegerid® in children.

Definitions/Abbreviations. Before going on and further discussing medications and reflux it would be best to define some of the terminology.

<u>Antacids.</u> Compounds that buffer stomach acid. Some are fast acting (sodium bicarbonate or $NaHCO_3$), some are slow acting (magnesium hydroxide or $MgOH_2$) and

some are intermediate acting (calcium carbonate or $CaCO_3$). Aluminum-containing antacids such as aluminum hydroxide are not very powerful in their ability to buffer acid. In addition, aluminum may accumulate in the body and may be linked to dementia. It also leads to constipation. Magnesium-containing antacids lead to looser stools.

Enteric-coated. A special coating that is put around a medicine so that it will not be destroyed by stomach acid. Enteric-coated medicines are usually absorbed into the blood stream just past the stomach, in the duodenum.

Esophagus. The tube that goes from the mouth to the stomach. When you swallow, food travels from your mouth to your stomach through the esophagus. This is also the part of your body that feels like it is burning when you get heartburn.

Evidence-Based Medicine. Making decisions about how to treat a patient based on good scientific studies. Nearly everyone in medicine today knows this term and claims to make decisions using evidence-based medicine. Unfortunately, most do not truly practice evidence-based medicine because it requires the scientific evidence to be read by the health-care provider and they simply do not have the time to do this. A few try and they are certainly worth seeking out. All of the information in this chapter is evidence-based.

Histamine type 2 receptor blockers (H-2RA, H-2 blocker). These medicines block histamine at the recep-

tor side of the parietal cell. H-2 blockers include cimetidine (Tagamet®), ranitidine (Zantac®®), famotidine
(Pepcid®), and nizatidine (Axid®).

Parietal cells. The cells that make stomach acid. Parietal
cells have a secreting end and a receptor end. Histamine is a chemical made by the body to bind to the receptor end of the parietal cell—this results in the stimula-
tion of the parietal cell. Parietal cells contain proton
pumps and, when stimulated, the proton pumps make
stomach acid (hydrochloric acid or HCL).

Pharmacokinetics. The study of the movement of medicines into, through, and out of the body.

Pharmacodynamics. The study of the actions of medicines upon the body; in other words, how the medicines
work in the body.

Pharmacology. The study of medicines.

Proton pumps. Proteins inside of the parietal cell that
trade hydrogen (H+) for potassium (K+). The proton
pumps concentrate the H+ to the outside of the cell
membrane and the K+ on the inside. The hydrogen (H+)
combines with chloride (Cl-) and you get stomach acid,
or HCl. The proton pumps represent the final step in
making stomach acid.

Proton pump inhibitor (PPI). Medicines that work by
blocking the proton pump's ability to trade H+ for K+.
PPIs include omeprazole (Prilosec®, Zegerid®), lanso-

prazole (Prevacid®), pantoprazole (Protonix®), rabeprazole (Aciphex®), and esomeprazole (Nexium®).

<u>Sucralfate.</u> The trade name is Carafate®. A medicine that
is a sticky sugar combined with aluminum that works by
binding to irritated places in the stomach lining or
esophagus. Sucralfate requires the presence of acid and
an irritation in the esophagus or stomach lining to work.
Once the irritation starts to heal the sucralfate does not
bind.

<u>Stomach acid.</u> Stomach acid is also called hydrochloric
acid (HCL) or gastric acid. It is a powerful acid that can
cause the destruction of the stomach wall, esophagus
wall, or wall of the small bowel (such as duodenum or
jejunum).

<u>Trade name/generic name.</u> Medicines have two names:
   1) The general chemical name that is used through-
      out the world is the generic name.
   2) The name that the company gives to the medicine
      is the trade name.

For example, omeprazole is a generic name and Pril-
osec® is the trade name for that mediation. Since the
patent protection has ended for omeprazole, the generic
form is also available by a different drug company. Trade
names are capitalized and have a TM or ® after the
name and generic names are not capitalized.

Drugs for GERD Treatment

Pharmacologic therapy that achieves effective control of intragastric pH reduces many of the typical as well as atypical signs and symptoms of gastroesophageal reflux disease.[5,8,13,17,29-34] The pharmacologic treatment of reflux disease in pediatric patients frequently includes the use of a prokinetic agent such as cisapride or metoclopramide* along with anti-acid secretory agents such as the histamine type 2 receptor antagonists, often with antacids and/or sucralfate. The use of these agents is most often only partially effective in relieving the symptoms of reflux and requires the caregiver to administer multiple agents numerous times per day.

PPIs, while highly effective in adult GERD, have been very slow to catch on in the pediatric community. In adults, PPIs are typically dosed once or twice daily. Still many adult patients complain of poor control of their GERD symptoms (especially at nighttime). In young children, these PPI drugs are not easy to use since many young children are unable to swallow the capsules or tablets. This would have seemed to have been alleviated with the introduction of Prevacid® SoluTabs and Prevacid® Delayed-Release Suspension; however, these medicines contain small granules that cannot be chewed or smashed. Very young children simply are unable to swallow these pellets, which contain the medicine. In addition, choking is a concern in such settings.

---

* Cisapride is no longer available because of fatal cardiac rhythm disturbances. Metoclopramide (Reglan®) causes significant behavioral abnormalities and has been evaluated over and over and found to provide little or no efficacy.

Medications for Acid Reflux

The main medications that are effective in treating acid reflux–related disorders in children either neutralize, block, or inhibit the effects of stomach acid.

Drugs that neutralize stomach acid.

Antacids. When the discomfort of reflux flares up due to acid irritating the esophagus, antacids can provide some relief (Figure 13-1). They work to **neutralize acid** in the stomach and raise the pH to a more neutral, comfortable level. Stomach acid naturally has an extremely low pH. It is considered an acid because of the high number of loose atoms (or ions) of hydrogen.

The body provides its own buffer, bicarbonate, to keep these ions under control. The bicarbonate chemically collects the loose hydrogen ions, neutralizing the acid. However, sometimes when there is an excess of hydrogen ions, what the body provides naturally isn't enough. Antacids act as an additional buffer to help collect extra hydrogen ions. Reflux may still occur, but the more neutral pH of the acid is far less irritating, helps in healing previous damage, and protects from further damage.

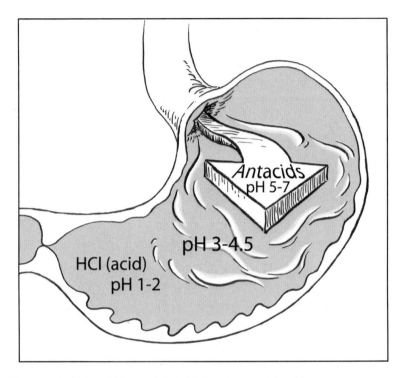

Figure 13-1. Antacids work by raising the gastric pH.

Antacids that contain magnesium and/or calcium work best for occasional use. Aluminum-containing antacids are weak and may lead to aluminum toxicity or dementia. Antacids are most useful when given occasionally, like in between doses of other drugs. A note to remember is that magnesium, which may be found in antacids, causes a loosening of stools. Table 13-1 list the strong and weak types of antacids. <u>IMPORTANT: If your child has kidney disease, do not use antacids without speaking to your medical doctor.</u>

Table 13-1. Types of antacids and their strengths

Antacids	weak	strong
Aluminum hydroxide	X	
Calcium carbonate		X
Magnesium hydroxide		X
Sodium bicarbonate		X

Some Antacid Recommendations. Maalox® Quick Dissolve chewable Extra Strength tablets in the wild berry flavor taste good and contain 1000 mg of calcium carbonate per tablet which is a good form of antacid for temporary relief of reflux symptoms. For small children (1 year and under) break one tablet into four equal pieces and dissolve one of the pieces in water or in the bottle of milk. For children 1 to 3 years, one half of a tablet can be used. Children 4 to 5 years and older can suck on one half to three fourths of a tablet. If you note that your child is having a lot of gas, then consider Maalox® Quick Dissolve Extra Strength with anti-gas. It contains 1000 mg of calcium carbonate per tablet and 60 mg simethicone (simethicone works to break up gas bubbles, making them easier to pass). Follow the above guidelines for dosage. A liquid form that tastes good is Mylanta® Supreme Cherry flavored liquid. It contains (in each 5 ml teaspoon) 400 mg of calcium carbonate and 135 mg of magnesium hydroxide. This is an especially good choice if your baby is having constipation or very hard and compact stools. For small children (under 1 year) give one half of a teaspoonful in a bottle of milk. For 1 to 3 years, three fourths to one teaspoonful can be used. For children 4 to 5 years and older give one teaspoonful.

NOTE: Only give your child a maximum of three doses of any antacid per day. If you need to use more than this, contact your doctor.

Sucralfate (Carafate®). Sucralfate is an aluminum-containing, sticky sugar that binds to open, irritated areas (ulcers) in the esophagus or stomach (Figure 13-2). Actually, sucralfate can be thought of as a Band-Aid® specifically for ulcers. Ulcers are crater-like injuries in the lining of the stomach, esophagus, or small intestine. The injury is the result of the presence of more irritants (e.g., stomach acid) than the stomach's own defense mechanisms can handle.

Once activated by stomach acid, sucralfate becomes a protective adherent paste that binds only to the ulcer. It prevents further damage by keeping hydrogen ions (acid) from seeping in, and promotes healing by enhancing the stomach's own line of self-defense. The catch is that sucralfate requires acid to become active. It also requires an irritated area. Because of these two factors, and since it has to be given quite frequently (4–6 times/day), it is not highly useful for the treatment of acid-related disorders in children.

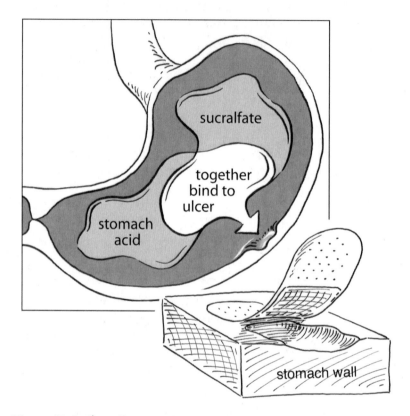

Figure 13-2. Sucralfate combines with stomach acid to protect and heal ulcers.

Sucralfate should not be used with antacids or with H-2 blockers or with PPI drugs. This is because sucralfate requires an acidic environment to work.

Drugs that block the production of stomach acid. In order to understand how these drugs work, it is helpful to understand how the body makes acid. The upper section of the gastrointestinal tract is made up of different parts (Figure 13-3). Acid is made in the walls of the stomach by cells known as parietal cells (Figure 13-4).

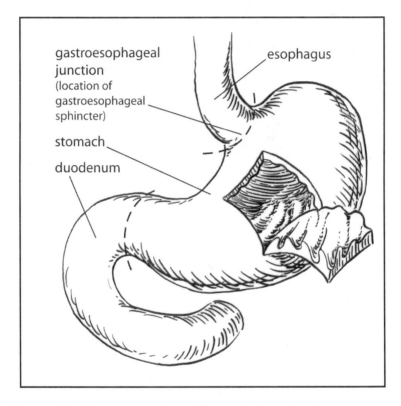

Figure 13-3. The upper section of the gastrointestinal tract.

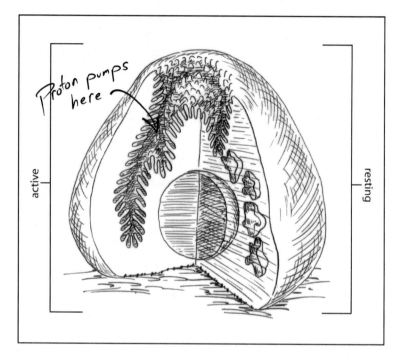

active

resting

Proton pumps here

Figure 13-4. A parietal cell.

The figure illustrates both states of a parietal cell at the same time. One side is active; the acid-making proton pumps are on. The other side is resting, not making much acid. When you eat, the parietal cells become more active, and in between eating they are less active. Also, in the early morning hours (2 A.M. to 6 A.M.) the parietal cells are actively making acid. Inside the wall of the stomach and working with the parietal cells are the G cells (gastrin making cells) and the ECL cells (making histamine). When food hits your stomach it causes the following to happen:

1) The G cells make and release gastrin.
2) The gastrin tells the ECL cells to make histamine
3) The histamine tells the parietal cell to make acid (by plugging into a receptor).

This turns on the proton pumps (acid pumps) that are inside the parietal cell. To put this process in perspec-

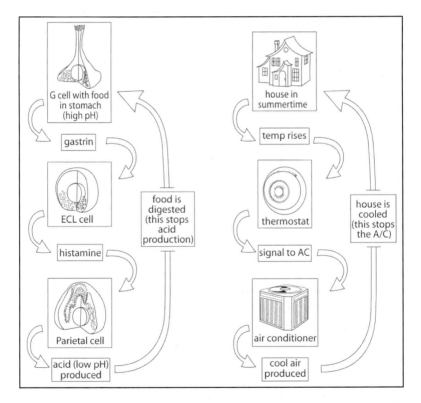

Figure 13-5. The acid making process compared to climate control.

tive, we can compare it to the way in which an air conditioner regulates temperature in a house (Figure 13-5).

<u>H-2 blockers</u>. Just after a meal, when the stomach is full, it tells the parietal cell to start acid production so that digestion can take place. The parietal cell gets the "go-ahead" from three different messengers, the major one being histamine (not to be confused with the histamine involved in allergies, which binds to a different receptor known as the H-1 receptor). Each messenger must locate its own specific receptor on the parietal cell wall to communicate with the cell. H-2 blockers stop the major messenger histamine from reaching its receptor (the H-2 receptor).The parietal cell can still get the go-ahead from the other two types of messengers, gastrin and muscarinic, but overall, acid production is significantly limited (Figure 13-6). (Please note that "H-2" may also be written as "H_2".)

The H-2 blockers are drugs such as Zantac® (ranitidine), Pepcid® (famotidine), Tagamet® (cimetidine), and Axid® (nizatidine). These drugs all work the same way: They block acid production by blocking the main receptor, the H-2 receptor, which is primarily responsible for turning on the parietal cells. There are two other receptors that can turn on the parietal cell; H-2 blockers only block the histamine type 2 receptors.

One of the problems with these drugs in children is that children develop tolerance (very rapidly) to the effects of all H-2 blockers. This can happen in as little as one week. You will know it is happening because your child

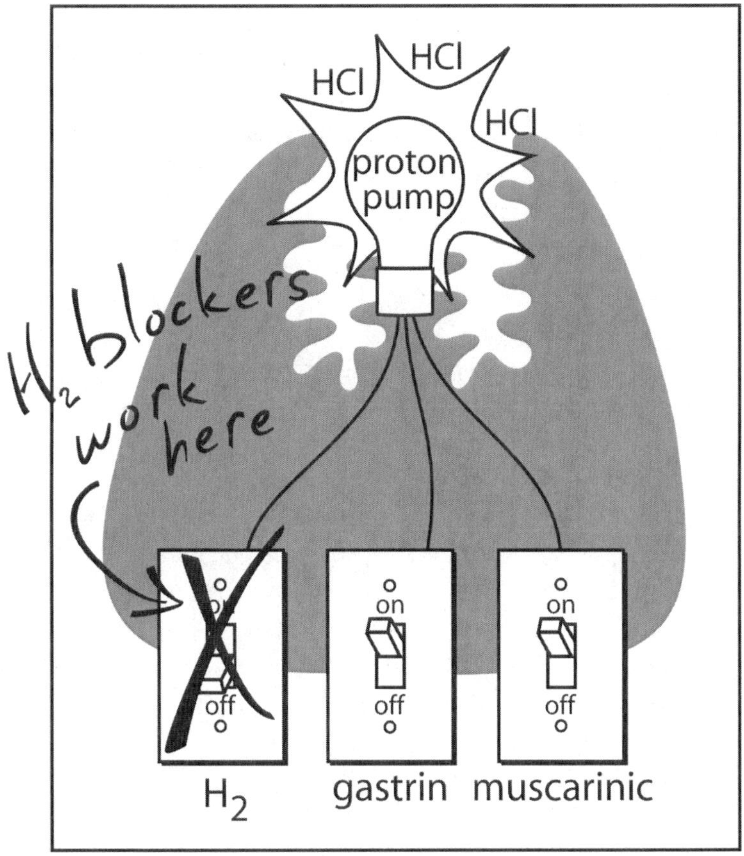

Figure 13-6. H-2 blockers work at the receptor end of the parietal cell.

will no longer feel good. In other words, he or she starts feeling good when you start the Zantac® or Pepcid® at the beginning, and then a week or so later the symptoms return. A special note—never use H-2 blockers along with PPI drugs. This is because the H-2 blocker will prevent the PPI drug from working. It is OK to give a PPI drug at breakfast and dinner and then four hours or more later, at bedtime, give an H-2 blocker. <u>But never give a PPI and an H-2 blocker at the same time.</u>

Generic and Trade Names for H-2 Blockers:
- Ranitidine (Zantac®)
- Famotidine (Pepcid®)
- Cimetidine (Tagamet®)
- Nizatidine (Axid®)

Drugs that inhibit the production of stomach acid.
<u>PPIs.</u> As described above, after a meal, when the stomach is full, it signals the parietal cell to start acid production so that digestion can take place. The real story though takes place on the surface of the parietal cell. This is where we find proton pumps busy pumping out stomach acid. These pumps are the source of stomach acid, and are therefore the target of the PPI, the proton pump inhibitor. The PPI binds to the proton pump and irreversibly stops it (Figure 13-7).

The catch, though, is that the PPI can inhibit only active proton pumps. So for the PPI to work at its best, there must be as many pumps *actively pumping* as possible. There are always some pumps pumping, but the time to find the most active pumps is just after a meal. That's why it is important to coordinate a meal with PPI intake.

PPIs are the drugs of choice for treating acid-related disorders in children. They are highly effective with a very wide safety margin. The main problem is that they are often under-dosed in children (see PPI Dosing Information). Based on current research it has been found

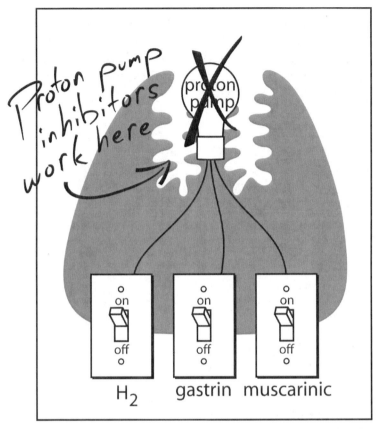

Figure 13-7. PPIs work at the acid-secreting end of the parietal cell.

that children metabolize PPI drugs about three times faster than adults and as such they require the drug to be given about three times per day to make up for the rapid elimination. Prilosec® (omeprazole), Nexium® (esomeprazole), and Prevacid® (lansoprazole) are enteric-coated, tiny granules that require a longer period of time to be effective. A new liquid product, Zegerid®, is available which contains omeprazole in a true suspension. This makes it much easier to use in very young children who are not yet taking solids. Prevacid® De-layed-Release suspension contains enteric-coated gran-ules and does not go into a true suspension. Note: The small pellets or granules must not be crushed or they will become ineffective.

PPIs are safer and more effective than H-2 blocker drugs. Children do not develop tolerance to the PPI drugs like they do to the H-2 blocker drugs. We use PPI drugs as standard treatment because PPIs are the saf-est, most effective medications available for treating acid reflux–related disorders in children and infants. The only PPIs currently approved by the FDA for pediatric use are lansoprazole and omeprazole.

Generic and Trade Names for PPIs:
- Lansoprazole (Prevacid®)
- Omeprazole (Prilosec®)
- Esomeprazole (Nexium®)
- Pantoprazole (Protonix®)
- Rabeprazole (Aciphex®)
- Omeprazole + buffer (Zegerid®)

PPI Dosing (In a Nutshell). Children need to get more doses per day of the PPI drugs because they eliminate the drugs so quickly. The elimination is measured and reported as half-life (t ½). Most children have a half-life of 27 minutes for PPIs whereas adults have a half-life of PPIs that is 80 minutes. So children eliminate the PPI drugs approximately three times faster than adults. Adults take the PPI drugs once per day, and many still complain of nighttime breakthrough of symptoms and then take the PPI twice per day. Therefore: 3 x (1) = 3 times per day for children. We have published our findings, which support that children need their PPI dose three times per day or sometimes four times per day. It is very simple math and basic pharmacokinetics.

The following may be more information than you need, but read on those of you who are math lovers. The way that a scientist can predict the effect that a PPI drug will have in blocking acid is by measuring the AUC (area under the curve). It is really quite simple to measure the AUC. You give a patient a dose of the PPI and then you start taking a little blood (from a vein of that patient) every few minutes and record the amount of the drug remaining in the blood stream. What you end up with is something like figure 13-8, a graph for a five month-old patient we will call BB.

In this case the AUC is the area under the line which we can calculate. The back part of the curve (where the arrow is pointing) is used to determine the half-life (how fast the drug is being eliminated).

The AUC is calculated as follows:

$$AUC = \frac{Dose \times t\frac{1}{2}}{Vd\ (0.693)}$$

Studies performed and published to date have shown that children have a shorter t ½ (half-life) than adults and a larger Vd (volume of distribution). A larger Vd dictates that a larger dose be given and a shorter t ½ dictates that the dose be give more often. In general, the half-life is three times faster than the adult and the Vd is three to four times larger than the adult (on a mg/k basis). Based upon these differences, Tables 13-2 and 13-3 list the appropriate pediatric dosages for lansoprazole and omeprazole.

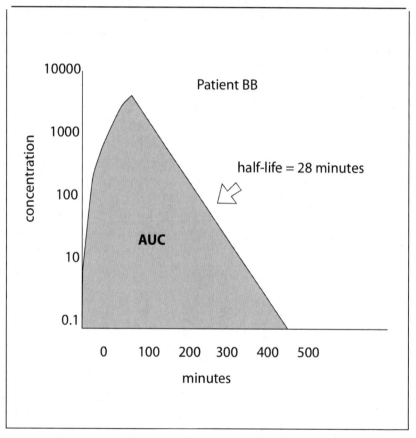

Figure 13-8. PPI half-life in 5-month-old patient BB.

The following are dosing recommendations for pediatric patients and are based upon the research and usage of the MARCI-Kids team (www.marci-kids.com) at the University of Missouri. In some children, a higher or a lower dose is required to control symptoms. These recommendations are designed to be a starting place to assist your physician in choosing the right dose for your child. **Your physician must make the decision on choosing medicines and doses for your child.**

Table 13-2. Pediatric Dosing for Lansoprazole

Dosing dependent on age and weight

Age	Dose per day (mg/kg)
< 3 months	1.5 to 1.75 mg/kg three times per day
3 to 6 months	1.25 to 1.5 mg/mg three times per day
7 months to 2 years	1 to 1.25 mg/kg three times per day
> 2 years	1 mg/kg two or three times per day
> 5 years	0.75 to 1 mg/kg two times per day

Table 13-3. Pediatric Dosing for Omeprazole
Dosing dependent on age and weight

Age	Dose per day (mg/kg)
< 3 months	1.5 mg/kg three times per day
3 to 6 months	1.25 mg/kg three times per day
7 months to 2 years	1 mg/kg three times per day
> 2 years	1 mg/kg two or three times per day
> 5 years	0.75 to 1 mg/kg two times per day

Drugs that promote movement of contents through the stomach
Pro-Motility Drugs. Pro-motility drugs work to relieve two conditions often associated with reflux disorders:

1) delayed gastric emptying
2) a weak LES (lower esophageal sphincter)

In delayed gastric emptying, the stomach contents do not move through as quickly as they should, building excess pressure in the stomach. The LES is the valve between the esophagus and stomach. A weak LES will more likely give way to the excess pressure within the stomach, allowing the contents to reflux into the esophagus. Pro-motility drugs work on the nerves that control the muscles of the stomach. They strengthen the LES and get the stomach contents moving into the small intestine at a healthier pace.

Metoclopramide and cisapride are supposed to work by enhancing the emptying of the stomach and therefore are known as pro-motility or pro-kinetic agents. They have marginal efficacy and serious side-effect potential. The best available medical studies and reviews of studies reveal that these drugs are rarely if ever useful. They usually get prescribed because the PPI drug being used is not being dosed properly.

Metoclopramide has caused shaking and jerking movements, and sometimes rigid body posturing (acute dystonic reactions), which are often mistaken for seizures and can cause profound irritability and tiredness. Cisapride (Propulsid®) has caused fatal arrythmias in children and has low efficacy. The best studies available and independent reviews of studies of cisapride have shown its low efficacy.

Generic and Trade Names for Motility Drugs:
- Metoclopramide (Reglan®)
- Cisapride (Propulsid®)

Conclusion

Medications have a very specific and oftentimes beneficial use in treating patients, especially young patients, who may have acid reflux. Selection of the proper medication and the proper dosage of that medication are critical to successful treatment if medication is recommended.

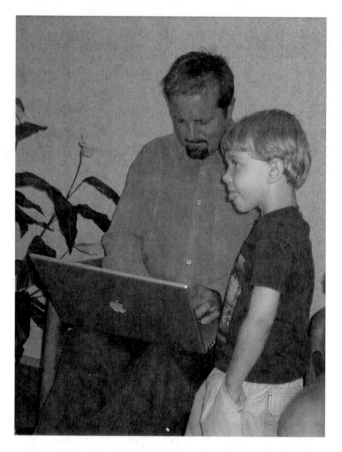

Co-author Dr. Jeffrey Phillips with Ben.

References

1. Mathews, B.L., J.P., Little, McGuirt, W.F., Jr., and J.A. Koufman. Reflux in infants with laryngomalacia: results of 24-hour double-probe pH monitoring. *Otolaryngol Head Neck Surg* 120 (June, 1999): 860-4.

2. Nelson, S., E. Chen, G. Syniar, and K. Christoffel. Prevalence of symptoms of gastroesophageal reflux during infancy: a pediatric practice-based survey. *Arch Pediatr Adolesc Med* 151 (Jun 1997): 569-72.

3. Tolaymat. N., and D.M. Chaptman. Gastroesophageal reflux disease in children older than two years of age. *The West Virginia Medical Journal* 94 (Jan-Feb 1998): 22-5.

4. Hodgman, J.E., F. Gonzales, T. Hoppenbrouwers, and L.A. Cabal. Apnea, transient episodes of bradycardia, and periodic breathing in preterm infants. *Am J Dis Child* 144 (Jan 1990): 54-7.

5. Andze, G.O., M.L. Brant, D. St. Vil, L.A. Bensoussan, and H. Blanchard. Diagnosis and treatment of gastroesophageal reflux in children with respiratory symptoms: The value of pH monitoring. *J Ped Surg* 26 (1991) 295-300.

6. Waki E.Y., D.N. Madgy, W.M. Belenky, and V.C. Gower. The incidence of gastroesophageal reflux in recurrent croup. *Int J Pediatr Otorhino-laryngol* 32 (Jul 1995): 223-32.

7. Danus, OI, C. Casar, A. Larrain, and C.E. Pope. Esophageal reflux—An unrecognized cause of recurrent obstructive bronchitis in children. *J of Ped* 89 (Aug 1976): 220-4.

8. Berquist, W.E., G.S. Rachelefsky, M. Kadden, S.C. Siegel, R.M. Katz, E.W. Fonkalsrud, and M.E. Ament. Gastroesophageal reflux associated recurrent pneumonia and chronic asthma in children. *Pediatrics* 68 (Jul 1981): 29-3.

9. Hampton FJ, CS MacFadyen, Beardsmore, H Simpson. Gastro-oesophageal reflux and respiratory function in infants with respiratory symptoms. *Arch of Dis Childhood* 66 (Jul 1991): 848-853.

10. Sheikh S, LJ Goldsmith, L Howell, J Hamlyn, N, Eid. Lung function in infants with wheezing and gastroesophageal reflux. *Ped Pulmonology* 27 (Apr 1999): 236-41.

11. Martin M.E., M.M. Grunstein, and G. Larsen. The relationship of gastroesophageal reflux to nocturnal wheezing in children with asthma. *Ann of Allergy* 49 (Dec 1982): 318-322.

12. Gumpert L, N. Kalach, C. Dupont, and P. Contencin. Hoarseness and gastroesophageal reflux in children. *J Laryngol and Otol* 112 (Jan 1998): 49-54.

13. Buts J.P., C. Barudi, D. Moulin, D. Claus, G. Cornu, J.B. Otte. Prevalence and treatment of silent gastro-oesophageal reflux in children with recurrent respiratory disorders. *Euro J Ped* 145 (Oct 1986): 396-400.

14. Euler A.R., W.J. Byrne, M.E. Ament, E.W. Fonkalsrud, C.T. Strobel, S.C. Siegel, R.M. Katz, and G.S. Rachelefsky. Recurrent pulmonary disease in children: A complication of gastroesophageal reflux. *Pediatrics* 63 (Jan 1979): 47-51.

15. Baer M., M. Maki, J. Nurminen, V. Turjanmaa, J. Pukander, and T. Vesikari. Esophagitis and findings of long-term esophageal pH recordings in children with repeated lower respiratory tract symptoms. *J Ped Gastroenterol and Nutr* 5 (Mar 1986): 187-190.

16. Shapiro G.G, and D.L. Christie. Gastroesophageal reflux in steroid-dependent asthmatic youths. *Pediatrics* 63 (Feb 1979): 207-211.

17. Tucci F., M. Resti, R. Fontana, E. Novembre, C.A. Lami, and A. Vierucci. Gastroesophageal reflux and bronchial asthma: Prevalence and effect of cisapride therapy. *J of Ped Gastroenterol and Nutr* 17 (Oct 1993): 265-270.

18. Giannoni C., M, Sulek, E.M. Friedman, and N.O. Duncan. Gastroesophageal reflux associated with laryngomalacia: A prospective study. *Intern J of Ped Otorhinolaryngology* 43 (Feb 1998): 11-20.

19. Belmont J.R., and K. Grundfast. Congenital laryngeal stridor (laryngomalacia): etiologic factors and associated disorders. *Annals of Otology, Rhinology and Laryngology* 93 (Sep-Oct 1984): 430-436.

20. Contencin P, and P. Narcy. Nasopharyngeal pH monitoring in infants and children with chronic rhinopharyngitis. *Intl J of Ped Otorhinolaryngol* 22 (Oct 1991): 249-56.

21. Walner D.L., Y. Stern, M.E. Gerber, C. Rudolph, C.Y. Baldwin, and R.T. Cotton. Gastroesophageal reflux in patients with sub-

glottic stenosis. *Arch Otolaryngology Head and Neck Surg* 124 (May 1998): 551-555.

22. Yellon R.F., M. Parameswaran, and B.W. Brandom. Decreasing morbidity following laryngotracheal reconstruction in children. *Intl J of Ped Otorhinolaryngol* 41 (Aug 1997): 145-154.

23. Gray C, F. Davies, and E. Molyneux. Apparent life-threatening events presenting to a pediatric emergency department. *Pediatr Emerg Care* 15 (Jun 1999): 195-199.

24. Marcus C.L. and A. Hamer. Significance of isolated bradycardia detected by home monitoring. *J Pediatr* 136 (Sep 1999): 321-326.

25. Meny R.G., J.L. Carroll, M.T. Carbone, and D.H. Kelly. Cardiorespiratory recordings from infants dying suddenly and unexpectedly at home. *Pediatrics* 93 (Jun 1994): 44-49.

26. Livera L.N., S.A. Spencer, M.S. Thorniley, Y.A. Wickramasinghe, and P. Rolfe. Effects of hypoxaemia and bradycardia on neonatal cerebral hemodynamics. *Arch Dis Child* 66 (1991): 376-380.

27. Kahn A, J. Riazi, and D. Blum. Oculocardiac reflux in near miss for sudden infant death syndrome infants. *Pediatrics* 71 (1983): 49-52.

28. Rahilly P.M.. The pneumographic and medical investigation of infants suffering apparent life threatening episodes. *J Paediatr Child Health* 27 (Dec 1991): 349-353.

29. Herbst J.J., S.D. Minton, and L.S. Book. Gastroesophageal reflux causing respiratory distress and apnea in newborn infants. *J of Ped* 95 (Nov 1979): 763-768.

30. Hof E., J. Hirsing, A. Giedion, and J.P. Pochon. Deleterious consequences of gastroesophageal reflux in cleft laryngeal surgery. *J of Ped Surg* 22 (1987): 197-19.

31. Halstead L.A.. Gastroesophageal reflux: A critical factor in pediatric subglottic stenosis. *Otolaryngology – Head and Neck Surgery* 120 (May 1999): 683-688.

32. Gibson WS, and W. Cochran. Otalgia in infants and children–A manifestation of gastroesophageal reflux. *Intl J Ped Otorhinolaryngol* 28 (Jan 1994): 213-218.

33. Jolley S.G., J.J. Jerbst, D.G. Johnson, M.E. Matlak, and L.S. Book. Surgery in children with gastroesophageal reflux and respiratory symptoms. *J of Ped* 96 (Feb 1980): 194-198.

34. Gustafsson P.M., N.-IM. Kjellman, L. Tibbling. A trial of ranitidine in asthmatic children and adolescents with or without pathological gastro-oesophageal reflux. *Eur Resp J* 5 (Feb 1992): 201-206.

35. Vigneri S, R. Termini, G. Leandro, et al. A comparison of five maintenance therapies for reflux esophagitis. *N Engl J Med* 333 (Oct 1995): 1106-1110.

36. Burget D.W., G. Stephen, S.G. Chiverton, and R.H. Hunt. Is there an optimal degree of acid suppression for healing of duodenal ulcer? A model of the relationship between ulcer healing and acid suppression. *Gastroenterol* 99 (1990): 345-351.

37. Bell NJ, D. Burget, C. Howden,. Appropriate acid suppression for the management of gastro-oesophageal reflux disease. *Digestion*: 51 (Suppl 1, 1992): 59-67.

38. Chiba N., C.J. De Gara, J.M. Wilkinson and R.H. Hunt,. Speed of healing and symptom relief in grade II to IV gastroesophageal reflux disease: A meta-analysis. *Gastroenterol* 112 (Jun 1997): 1798-1810.

39. Chun A.H.C., C.J. Eason, H.H. Shi, and J.H. Cavanaugh. Lansoprazole: An alternative method of administration of a capsule dosage formulation. *Clin Ther* 17 (May-Jun 1995): 441-447.

40. Chun A.H.C., H.H. Shi, R. Achari, S. Dennis, and J.H. Cavanaugh. Lansoprazole: Administration of the contents of a capsule dosage formulation through a nasogastric tube. *Clin Ther* 18 (Sep-Oct 1996): 833-842.

41. Sharma V.K., E.A. Ugheoke, R. Vasudeva, and C.W. Howden. The pharmacodynamics of lansoprazole administered via gastrostomy as intact, non-encapsulated granules. *Aliment Pharmacol Ther* 12 (Nov 1998): 1171-1174.

42. Zimmermann A., J.K. Walters, B. Katona, and P. Souney. Alternative methods of proton pump inhibitor administration. *Consult Pharm* 12 (Dec 1997): 990-998.

43. Sharma V.K., E.A. Ugheoke, R. Vasudeva, and C.W. Howden. Lansoprazole effectively suppresses intragastric acidity when administered via gastrostomy as intact granules in orange juice. *Gastroenterol* 114 (1998): A283.

44. Sharma V.K., R. Vasudeva, and C.W. Howden. Simplified lansoprazole suspension (SLS): A proton pump inhibitor (PPI) in a liquid formulation that works. *Am J Gastroenterol* 93 (1998): A1647.

45. Phillips J., and M. Metzler. Simplified omeprazole solution for the prophylaxis of stress-related mucosal damage in critically ill patients. *Crit Care Med* 22 (1994): A53.

46. Phillips J., M. Metzler, T.L. Palmieri, et al. A prospective study of simplified omeprazole suspension for the prophylaxis of stress-related mucosal damage. *Crit Care Med* 24 (Nov 1996): 1793-1780.

47. Phillips J., M. Metzler, R. Huckfeldt, and K. Olsen. A multicenter, prospective, randomized clinical trial of continuous infusion IV ranitidine vs. omeprazole suspension in the prophylaxis of stress ulcers. *Crit Care Med* 26 (1998): A101.

48. Lasky M., M. Metzler, and J. Phillips. A prospective study of omeprazole suspension to prevent clinically significant gastrointestinal bleeding from stress ulcers in mechanically ventilated trauma patients. *J of Trauma* 44 (Mar 1998): 527-53.

49. Kazuhide W., N. Matsuka, K. Furuno, K. Eto, H. Kawasaki, and Y. Gomita. Pharmacokinetic evaluation of omeprazole suspension following oral administration in rats: effect of neutralization of gastric acid. *Acta Med Okayama* 50 (Aug 1996): 219-22.

50. Phillips J.O., and M.H. Metzler. The stability of simplified lansoprazole suspension (SLS). *Gastroenterol* : 116 (suppl 1999): A89.

51. Gunasekaran T.S., and E.G. Hassall. Efficacy and safety of omeprazole for severe Gastroesophageal reflux in children. *J Pediatr* 123 (Jul 1993): 148-154.

52. Hassall E., R. Shepaherd, M. Radke, A. Dalvag, O. Junghard, and P. Lundborg. Omeprazole for chronic erosive esophagitis in children: A multicenter study of dose requirement for healing. *Gastroenterol* 112 (suppl 1997): A425.

53. Israel D.M., and E. Hassall. Omeprazole and other proton pump inhibitors: pharmacology, efficacy, and safety with special reference to use in children. *J Pediatr Gastroenterol Nutr* 27 (1998): 568-79.

AFTERWORD

It's Not Over Until It's Over

D r. Jeff Phillips, who co-wrote Chapter 13, once told us, "Reflux comes in waves." One of the things that has become very clear to us about reflux is that it's not over until it's over.

We found that just about the time that Ben would adjust to a new medication, it would stop working, or just about the time that a new medication would appear to have the reflux and nighttime choking under control, he would appear to be having seizure-type episodes each time he fell asleep. It then seemed that once his medication would be under control, he would begin cutting teeth, or even worse, contract the rotavirus, and let's not even mention the introduction of solid food and the associated repercussions. Now, as an older child, defining his safe food zone has also been challenging.

Hopefully, this won't be your situation, but we do want you to be aware ahead of time that some days you may feel like you have conquered all, just to find out that the constant acid baths have caused an enormous amount of erosion on your baby's new teeth, or that the continuous reflux is creating numerous ear infections.

Patience Is Definitely Going to Be Needed

While a lot has been learned about treating reflux, there is no cure, and there really isn't always a complete understanding of what the disease is. Your final treatment may involve some art versus science—the solution may be 80% science, and the last 20% may be art. This is one of the reasons that you want to work with someone with a lot of reflux knowledge and experience: to improve the art part. Because art is involved it requires patience. For example, Ben had a reaction to two very common medications and that required several doctors to experiment with dosages and medications. That took months to perfect (unlike, say, a sinus infection for which you can almost always count on a single prescription of medication to do the trick).

You Must Be Vigilant

As the caregiver, you are closest to your child, which means that you must be vigilant, even though this thing may go on for a while longer than you had hoped. And there are three aspects to vigilance.

First, changes to your child's health can be subtle and can happen almost unbeknownst to you. These changes may come in the form of the baby waking up three times a night, then four times, and before you know it you are back to being up 12 times a night because your child has just been through a growth spurt and has outgrown the present dosage of medication.

Second, since you are the one closest to your child, you will be in a position to see things that your healthcare provider won't be able to see.

Third, you know the complete history of your child and can be the one to connect the dots others might not. For instance, even if the reflux is well treated, or even if it is resolved, there may be lingering issues.

Physically, there could be issues, such as tooth decay. For example research has shown that reflux can cause severe damage to teeth. As one author noted, "Intrinsic erosion is especially damaging since gastric acids are shown to be three times more erosive to tooth structure than the phosphoric acids found in soft drinks."[1]

Psychologically, there could be issues. Acid reflux can predispose children to have negative expectations about their world.[2] An infant who struggled through eating due to reflux may develop into a toddler who finds meal time stressful.

Developmentally, issues may also appear in areas such as speech, and it may even be that infants and young children with significant reflux may be more prone to some degree of language difficulties.

Endurance

No matter what the complexity, pediatric gastroesophageal reflux is an endurance test for the entire family. Because the challenges seem to just keep on coming, it might be a good idea to enlist the help of a therapist. We have found a great guy who has the experience of someone in his family being sick, and knows the day-to-day pressure that situation can create.

We have asked him very specifically to be a part of Ben's treatment team, by helping us not only to keep our anxiety in check, but also to give us the strength and encouragement to go the extra mile to get Ben the best care we can manage. He was key in supporting our initial trip to the University of Missouri, which made a huge difference in the quality of Ben's life). This has involved meeting with him every few weeks and going over what has transpired with Ben, including any medical test results. This helps us remain on an emotional even keel, keep things in perspective, and have the emotional strength to be proactive.

Current research suggests that many affected children outgrow most or all of their symptoms of reflux between the ages of 1 and 5 years.[3] However, you don't know when that might happen for your child. It could be one year, it could be five years, or it could be never. As Dr. Wirtz said in his chapter, caring for someone with a chronic illness is a lot like running a marathon, except in the case of reflux, you don't know when the finish line will appear (and if it ever will).

The Power of You

Jon Kabat-Zinn, in his book *Full Catastrophe Living*, writes:

> There is an art to facing difficulties in ways that lead to effective solutions. When we are able to mobilize our inner resources to face our problems artfully, we find we are usually able to orient ourselves in such a way that we can use the pressure of the problem itself to propel us through it, just as a sailor can position a sail to make the best use of the pressure of the wind to propel itself.[4]

This may be a long haul for you and your family. You are the one that can make the greatest difference in the quality of life for your child, your family, and you. According to Dr. Sears,

> I mention to parents that it is important for them to feel like valuable members of the medical team, because the treatment of GER is primarily parental intensive care. That is an important message that parents need to understand. GER is not anything that any medicine is completely going to fix.[5]

Chronic pain demands a proactive mind-set. You need to help yourself at a time when all you want is for someone to save you. Believe in yourself, and trust your instincts. If you think that something is wrong with your child, don't give up, and believe in the power of you.

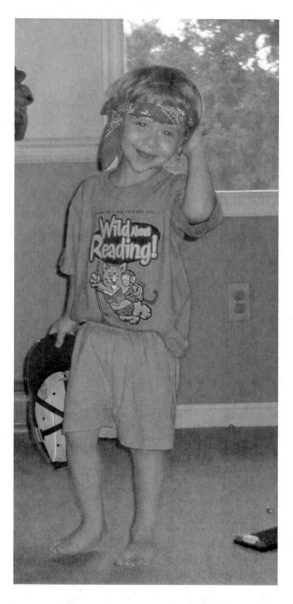

Making Life Better for a Child with Acid Reflux

1. Shipley, S., K. Taylor, and W. Mitchell. Identifying causes of dental erosion. *General Dentistry.* (Jan–Feb, 2004): 73-5.

2. Thyre, S.M. Mothers' internal working models with infants with gastroesophageal reflux. *Maternal-Child Nursing Journal* 22, 2 (1994): 39-48.

3. Hu F.Z., R.A. Preston, J.C. Post, G.J. White, L.W. Kikuchi, X. Wang, S.M. Leal, M.A. Levenstien, J. Ott, T.W. Self, G. Allen, R.S. Stiffler, C. McGraw, E.A. Pulsifer-Anderson, and G.D. Ehrlich. Mapping of a gene for severe pediatric gastroesophageal reflux to chromosome 13q14. *Journal of the American Medical Association* 284 (Jul 2000): 325-34.

4. Eating problems and reflux—part II, home intervention. *Reflux Digest* 5;1 (Spring/Summer 2001): 11.

5. Interview with Bill Sears, M.D. *Reflux Digest* 6;1 (Summer 2002): 4

APPENDIX A

RESOURCES

Where do you—where can you—turn for more information? Information that you can trust and hopefully will be helpful?

To answer that we have included a list of resources here that we have used, and found to be useful. Additionally, resources are listed at the end of many of the specific chapters in the book. One word to the wise, you will notice that the following are all web sites. Before you place any value on information that you find keep in mind that your own medical team is your best source of information (should be) and your most trusted source (has to be).

About Reflux and children

http://aboutkidsgi.org/gerd.html

http://www.aboutgerd.org

http://www.digestive.nlddk.nih.ogv/ddiseases/pubs/gerd/

http://www.forparentsbyparents.com

http://www.healingwell.com

http://www.healthcentral.com/acid-reflux/websites.html

http://www.infant-reflux.com

http://www.infantreflux.org

http://www.infantrefluxdisease.com

http://www.kidsacidreflux.org

http://www.marcikids.org

http://www.nocolic.com

http://www.reflux.org

Other Information

The Food Allergy and Anaphylaxis Network (FAAN)
11781 Lee Jackson Highway, Suite 160
Fairfax, VA 22033-3309
(800)929-4040

FAAN provides *The Food Allergy News Cookbook*

Food Allergy Field Guide – A Lifestyle Manual for Families by Theresa Willingham. Savory Palate, Inc. 2000.

Mead Johnson Nutritionals
Customer Service   1-800-457-3550
Website   www.meadjohnson.com

Ross Products
Customer Service   1-800-258-7677
Website   www.Ross.com

Nestle
Customer Service   1-800-422-2752
Website   www.NestleClinicalNutrition.com

SHS North America   1-800-365-7354
Website   www.neocateusa.com

ACKNOWLEDGEMENTS

Thanks to all of the contributors who volunteered their time to make this book a great resource for many: to our friends and family for keeping us laughing throughout the process of writing the book; to our editor, Robyn Alvarez for making us cry with all her red marks; to our babysitters Chelsea Prior and Ashley Smith for hanging with the boys while we tried to make sense of it all; to Nick Kovijanic and Claire Shipman for their early reviews; to Zane and Nancy Carter for their great support and wisdom; and to Benjamin's medical team of Susan Bauer, Marcella Bothwell, the folks at Edward's Pharmacy, Andrew Ferguson, Michele Innes, Stephen Latimer, Jeffrey Phillips, Mary Sahinci, Patrick Shanahan, Richard Wirtz, and Robert Wood for making life better for a child with acid reflux.

INDEX

Comments Please

How did you like this book? Was it helpful? Want to tell others about it? We're looking for endorsements and testimonials. If you have any you would like to share, let us know. Your help is greatly appreciated. Endorsements usually appear in the following year's edition.

Just fill out the info below, and send off to:

SportWork
Main Street
PO Box 102
Church Hill, MD 21623
(410) 556-6030 (p/f)
tracy@refluxguide.com

Name:		
Address:		
City:	State	Zip:
E-mail:		
Comments:		

Information Update Form

Your feedback is very important to help make this book a better product. If you have information you would like to share, or notice areas of this book that can be improved, let us know.

Just fill out the info below, and send off to:

SportWork
PO Box 102
Main Street
Church Hill, MD 21623
(410) 556-6030 (p/f)
tracy@refluxguide.com

Your help is greatly appreciated. Corrections to the text usually appear in the following year's edition.

Name:		
Address:		
City:	State	Zip:
E-mail:		
Comments:		

Quick Order Form

STEP 1: Grab a pen/pencil; **STEP 2:** Complete all information below; **STEP 3:** Mail this form and payment (check / purchase order) to: *SportWork, Main Street, PO Box 192, Church Hill, MD 21623.* (Orders may also be placed at www.refluxguide.com.)

Shipping Information

Name:	
Organization:	
Address:	
Address:	
City:	State:	Zip:
Phone:	E-mail:

Ordering Information

	Quantity	Price	Total
	_____	@ $19.95	_____
		Quantity Discount (see below)	_____
		Shipping (free within US, others contact us at 410-556-6030)	
		Tax (5% for MD residents)	_____
		Total (prepayment required, pay by credit card at Website)	_____

Acid Reflux in Infants and Children

Discounts:
3–11 books: 20% off retail price
12–36 books: 40% off retail price
37 books and up: 55% off retail price

244